Everyday Ethics in the Clinical Practice of Pediatrics and Young Adult Medicine

Editor

MARGARET R. MOON

PEDIATRIC CLINICS
OF NORTH AMERICA

www.pediatric.theclinics.com

Consulting Editor
TINA L. CHENG

February 2024 • Volume 71 • Number 1

ELSEVIER

1600 John F. Kennedy Boulevard • Suite 1800 • Philadelphia, Pennsylvania, 19103-2899

http://www.theclinics.com

THE PEDIATRIC CLINICS OF NORTH AMERICA Volume 71, Number 1
February 2024 ISSN 0031-3955, ISBN-13: 978-0-323-93929-4

Editor: Kerry Holland
Developmental Editor: Saswoti Nath

The Pediatric Clinics of North America (ISSN 0031-3955) is published bimonthly by Elsevier Inc., 360 Park Avenue South, New York, NY 10010-1710. Months of issue are February, April, June, August, October, and December. Periodicals postage paid at New York, NY and additional mailing offices. Subscription prices are $290.00 per year (US individuals), $368.00 per year (Canadian individuals), $440.00 per year (international individuals), $100.00 per year (US students and residents), $100.00 per year (Canadian students and residents), and $165.00 per year (international residents and students). For institutional access pricing please contact Customer Service via the contact information below. To receive students/resident rare, orders must be accompanied by name of affiliated institution, date of term, and the signature of program/residency coordinator on institution letterhead. Orders will be billed at individual rate until proof of status is received. Foreign air speed delivery is included in all *Clinics* subscription prices. All prices are subject to change without notice. **POSTMASTER:** Send address changes to *The Pediatric Clinics of North America*, Elsevier Health Sciences Division, Subscription Customer Service, 3251 Riverport Lane, Maryland Heights, MO 63043. **Customer Service: 1-800-654-2452 (US and Canada). From outside of the US and Canada: 1-314-447-8871. Fax: 1-314-447-8029. For print support, E-mail: JournalsCustomerService-usa@elsevier.com. For online support, E-mail: JournalsOnlineSupport-usa@elsevier.com.**

Reprints. For copies of 100 or more, of articles in this publication, please contact the Commercial Reprints Department, Elsevier Inc., 360 Park Avenue South, New York, NY 10010-1710. Tel.: 212-633-3874; Fax: 212-633-3820; E-mail: reprints@elsevier.com.

The Pediatric Clinics of North America is also published in Spanish by McGraw-Hill Inter-americana Editores S.A., Mexico City, Mexico; in Portuguese by Riechmann and Affonso Editores, Rua Comandante Coelho 1085, CEP 21250, Rio de Janeiro, Brazil; and in Greek by Althayia SA, Athens, Greece.

The Pediatric Clinics of North America is covered in *MEDLINE/PubMed (Index Medicus), Excerpta Medica, Current Contents, Current Contents/Clinical Medicine, Science Citation Index, ASCA, ISI/BIOMED,* and *BIOSIS*.

PROGRAM OBJECTIVE

The goal of the *Pediatric Clinics of North America* is to keep practicing physicians and residents up to date with current clinical practice in pediatrics by providing timely articles reviewing the state-of-the-art in patient care.

TARGET AUDIENCE

All practicing pediatricians, physicians, and healthcare professionals who provide patient care to pediatric patients.

LEARNING OBJECTIVES

Upon completion of this activity, participants will be able to:

1. Review barriers to cohesive goals of care, for children living with serious/complex medical conditions and strategies for addressing the challenges.
2. Discuss the pediatrician's valuable role in evaluating clinical ethics concerns.
3. Recognize ways in which pediatricians navigate challenges while attempting to simultaneously report and support children with medical complexities.

ACCREDITATIONS

Physician Credit

The Elsevier Office of Continuing Medical Education (EOCME) is accredited by the Accreditation Council for Continuing Medical Education (ACCME) to provide continuing medical education for physicians.

The EOCME designates this journal-based activity for a maximum of 10 *AMA PRA Category 1 Credit*(s)™. Physicians should claim only the credit commensurate with the extent of their participation in the activity.

All other healthcare professionals requesting continuing education credit for this journal-based activity will be issued a certificate of participation.

ABP Maintenance of Certification Credit

Successful completion of this CME activity, which includes participation in the activity and individual assessment of and feedback to the learner, enables the learner to earn up to 10 MOC points in the American Board of Pediatrics' (ABP) Maintenance of Certification (MOC) program. It is the CME activity provider's responsibility to submit learner completion information to ACCME for the purpose of granting ABP MOC credit.

DISCLOSURE OF CONFLICTS OF INTEREST

The EOCME assesses conflict of interest with its instructors, faculty, planners, and other individuals who are in a position to control the content of CME activities. All relevant conflicts of interest that are identified are thoroughly vetted by EOCME for fair balance, scientific objectivity, and patient care recommendations. EOCME is committed to providing its learners with CME activities that promote improvements or quality in healthcare and not a specific proprietary business or a commercial interest.

The planning committee, staff, authors, and editors listed below have identified no financial relationships or relationships to products or devices they or their spouse/life partner have with commercial interest related to the content of this CME activity:

Renee D. Boss, MD, MHS; Joseph A. Carrese, MD, MPH, FACP; Carrie M. Henderson, MD; D. Micah Hester, PhD; Mark T. Hughes, MD, MA, FACP, FAAHPM; Nicholas A. Jabre, MD, MS; Michelle Littlejohn; Rajkumar Mayakrishnan, BSc, MBA; Skye A. Miner, PhD; Margaret Moon, MD, MPH; Douglas J. Opel, MD, MPH; Mary A. Ott, MD, MA; Lainie Friedman Ross, MD, PhD; Kimberly E. Sawyer, MD, MA, HEC-C; Rebecca R. Seltzer, MD, MHS; B. Simone Thompson, LCSW-C

UNAPPROVED/OFF-LABEL USE DISCLOSURE

The EOCME requires CME faculty to disclose to the participants:

1. When products or procedures being discussed are off-label, unlabelled, experimental, and/or investigational (not US Food and Drug Administration [FDA] approved); and
2. Any limitations on the information presented, such as data that are preliminary or that represent ongoing research, interim analyses, and/or unsupported opinions. Faculty may discuss information about pharmaceutical agents that is outside of FDA-approved labelling. This information is intended solely for CME and is not intended to promote off-label use of these medications. If you have any questions, contact the medical affairs department of the manufacturer for the most recent prescribing information.

TO ENROLL

To enroll in the *Pediatric Clinics of North America* Continuing Medical Education program, call customer service at 1-800-654-2452 or sign up online at http://www.theclinics.com/home/cme. The CME program is available to subscribers for an additional annual fee of USD 313.00.

METHOD OF PARTICIPATION

In order to claim credit, participants must complete the following:

1. Complete enrolment as indicated above.
2. Read the activity.
3. Complete the CME Test and Evaluation. Participants must achieve a score of 70% on the test. All CME Tests and Evaluations must be completed online.

In order to claim MOC points, participants must complete the following:

1. Complete steps listed above for claiming CME credit
2. Provide your specialty board ID#, birth date (MM/DD), and attestation.
3. Online MOC submission is only available for the American Board of pediatrics' (ABP) Maintenance of Certification (MOC) program

CME INQUIRIES/SPECIAL NEEDS

For all CME inquiries or special needs, please contact elsevierCME@elsevier.com

Contributors

CONSULTING EDITOR

TINA L. CHENG, MD, MPH
BK Rachford Professor and Chair of Pediatrics, University of Cincinnati, Director, Cincinnati Children's Research Foundation, Chief Medical Officer, Cincinnati Children's Hospital Medical Center, Cincinnati, Ohio

EDITOR

MARGARET R. MOON, MD, MPH
Associate Professor of Pediatrics, Director, Department of Pediatrics, Pediatrician-in-Chief, Johns Hopkins School of Medicine, Co-Director, Johns Hopkins Children's Center, Core Faculty, The Johns Hopkins Berman Institute of Bioethics, Johns Hopkins University, Baltimore, Maryland

AUTHORS

RENEE D. BOSS, MD, MHS
Rembrandt Professor of Pediatric Palliative Care, Department of Pediatrics, Johns Hopkins School of Medicine, Johns Hopkins Berman Institute of Bioethics, Baltimore, Maryland

JOSEPH A. CARRESE, MD, MPH, FACP
Professor of Medicine, Division of General Internal Medicine, Johns Hopkins Bayview Medical Center, Core Faculty, Johns Hopkins Berman Institute of Bioethics, Johns Hopkins University, Baltimore, Maryland

CARRIE M. HENDERSON, MD
Professor, Department of Pediatrics, Center for Bioethics and Medical Humanities, University of Mississippi Medical Center, Jackson, Mississippi

D. MICAH HESTER, PhD
Professor, Chair, Department of Medical Humanities and Bioethics, College of Medicine, University of Arkansas for Medical Science, Little Rock, Arkansas

MARK T. HUGHES, MD, MA, FACP, FAAHPM
Assistant Professor of Medicine, General Internal Medicine, Core Faculty, Berman Institute of Bioethics, Johns Hopkins University School of Medicine, Baltimore, Maryland

NICHOLAS A. JABRE, MD, MS
Assistant Professor of Pediatrics, Johns Hopkins School of Medicine, Division of Pediatric Pulmonology, Johns Hopkins All Children's Hospital, St Petersburg, Florida

SKYE A. MINER, PhD
Assistant Professor, Department of Medical Humanities and Bioethics, College of Medicine, University of Arkansas for Medical Science, Little Rock, Arkansas

MARGARET R. MOON, MD, MPH
Associate Professor of Pediatrics, Director, Department of Pediatrics, Pediatrician-in-Chief, Johns Hopkins School of Medicine, Co-Director, Johns Hopkins Children's Center, Core Faculty, The Johns Hopkins Berman Institute of Bioethics, Johns Hopkins University, Baltimore, Maryland

DOUGLAS J. OPEL, MD, MPH
Professor, Department of Pediatrics, School of Medicine, University of Washington, Treuman Katz Center for Pediatric Bioethics, Interim Director, Seattle Children's Research Institute, Seattle, Washington

MARY A. OTT, MD, MA
Professor of Pediatrics, Adjunct Professor of Philosophy and Bioethics, Indiana University School of Medicine, Indianapolis, Indiana

LAINIE FRIEDMAN ROSS, MD, PhD
Dean's Professor and Chair, Department of Health Humanities and Bioethics, Professor, Department of Pediatrics, University of Rochester School of Medicine and Dentistry, Paul M. Schyve Center for Bioethics, Professor, Department of Philosophy, University of Rochester, Rochester, New York

KIMBERLY E. SAWYER, MD, MA, HEC-C
Assistant Professor, Department of Pediatrics, Baylor College of Medicine, Assistant Professor, Texas Children's Hospital Palliative Care Team, Houston, Texas

REBECCA R. SELTZER, MD, MHS
Department of Pediatrics, Johns Hopkins School of Medicine, Johns Hopkins Berman Institute of Bioethics, Department of Population, Family, and Reproductive Health, Johns Hopkins Bloomberg School of Public Health, Baltimore, Maryland

B. SIMONE THOMPSON, LCSW-C
Department of Pediatrics, Johns Hopkins Hospital, Baltimore, Maryland

Contents

> Clinical ethics is the dimension of bioethics devoted to analyzing competing values and obligations in clinical care, seeking the optimal balance between competing duties. Competence in clinical ethics is particularly important in our current scientific and social environment, where disharmony and challenges between value systems are common and the medical profession suffers from self-imposed risks to integrity and coherence. The ability to bring ethical analysis into the challenges of everyday clinical practice is a crucial component in resolving values conflicts and protecting the clinician–patient relationship that is the heart of our profession.

> Pediatricians have a fiduciary responsibility to advocate for the best interests of their patients. They accomplish this through the therapeutic alliance with the patient and their parent. In everyday clinical medicine, the pediatrician may be faced with challenging situations. When a case raises concerns, the pediatrician needs to determine if the issues relate to ethical obligations and whether they are in conflict. To resolve the concerns, a systematic process for gathering, organizing, and analyzing the facts of a case is needed to discern morally permissible options. This article presents a framework for performing an ethics case analysis.

> Although traditional medical ethics focuses on the dyadic doctor–patient relationship, when the patient is a child, the relationship is triadic, meaning it involves the patient, the parent(s), and the clinician. A brief examination of the family, the rights and responsibilities of parents, the rights of children, and the moral basis of the parent–child relationship provide a philosophic underpinning for understanding the family in pediatric decision-making. Although biological parents have presumptive authority to make health-care decisions for their children, and are given wide discretion, parental autonomy is not absolute.

Research involving pediatric populations has important ethical and regulatory considerations. As children generally cannot consent to research, there are special protections put in place to ensure that the decisional vulnerability is protected, including parental permission and often the child's assent. Assent is an ethically important part of the research because it allows the child to participate in the process of agreeing to research, develop their autonomy, and express their values. This article explores a case where the child and parent disagree about the child's participation. In doing so, the regulatory requirements of pediatric research are outlined and the process and product of obtaining assent from a minor is described.

Medicine is filled with uncertainty. Clinicians may experience uncertainty due to limitations in their own or existing medical knowledge. Uncertainty can be scientific, practical, or personal, and may involve issues related to probability, ambiguity, and complexity. Pediatricians face additional uncertainties related to the role of families in decision-making and limited ability to know the preferences of children. Clinicians may approach uncertainty in different ways: some choosing to embrace its presence and others attempting to avoid it. Ultimately, pediatricians must learn to navigate uncertainty together with their patients and families, minimizing it when possible while accepting that its presence is unavoidable.

This article presents three clinical scenarios that might be encountered in ambulatory pediatrics. The framework for ethical analysis presented by Dr Hughes in a separate article in this issue of the Journal is used to examine these clinical scenarios and demonstrate application of the framework. The three cases involve a physician being asked by parents to write a letter for better housing that would require the doctor to be dishonest; parents who decline to have their 8-month-old daughter vaccinated; and a physician who believes contraception is a sin and therefore would not prescribe it to a sexually active 17-year-old girl.

PEDIATRIC CLINICS OF NORTH AMERICA

Foreword
Everyday Ethics in a Changing World

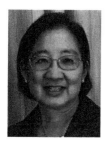

Tina L. Cheng, MD, MPH
Editor

Bioethics is defined as a "branch of applied ethics that studies the philosophic, social, and legal issues arising in medicine and the life sciences."[1] There is no shortage of philosophic, social, and legal issues that arise in our work as clinicians, researchers, educators, and child advocates. In this day and age of rapid scientific and technological advancement, ethical issues abound. Having a strong grounding in ethical principles and a framework to guide analysis can help navigate these issues.

There are unique issues in pediatric bioethics, including human reproduction and viability, the constantly growing and changing child, and adolescent development of autonomy, all ripe areas of bioethical discussion and debate. Bioethics often conjures memories of dramatic, headline-catching cases (eg, Baby Doe, Tuskegee syphilis study), but bioethical issues in pediatric practice are everyday issues. From my medical school training, I remember the 1979 Belmont Report's three principles of respect for persons, beneficence, and justice. Other principles of nonmaleficence, human dignity, and the sanctity of life can guide ethical analysis and moral decision making with further specification and balancing of these principles in specific cases.

Pediatr Clin N Am 71 (2024) xi–xii
https://doi.org/10.1016/j.pcl.2023.09.004
0031-3955/24/© 2023 Published by Elsevier Inc.

I am grateful to the authors in this issue, who offer frameworks and case studies to thoughtfully apply ethical principles in practice. These frameworks are critical, as new ethical issues continue to arise and as society and the practice of pediatrics evolve.

Tina L. Cheng, MD, MPH
Cincinnati Children's Hospital Medical Center
Cincinnati Children's Research Foundation
University of Cincinnati
3333 Burnet Avenue, MLC 3016
Cincinnati, OH 45229-3026, USA

E-mail address:
Tina.cheng@cchmc.org

REFERENCES

1. Britannica. Bioethics. Available at: https://www.britannica.com/topic/bioethics. Accessed September 15, 2023.

Preface

Everyday Ethics in the Clinical Practice of Pediatrics

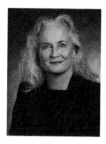

Margaret R. Moon, MD, MPH
Editor

Ethics is a method for analyzing conflicting moral obligations, seeking to identify the set of options that offers the best balance of obligations and a morally justifiable path forward. Clinical ethics has long been part of clinical practice, but the history of clinical ethics has tended to direct focus to dilemmas arising at the extremes of life, issues related to innovative technologies that challenge our understanding of life and death, or essential conflicts arising from nonmainstream religious or cultural beliefs. The field of clinical ethics owes much to the analyses of these extraordinary dilemmas; they have identified boundaries of rights and responsibilities, created paradigms for interpretation and methods for review, defined curricula for clinical education, pushed policy and advocacy forward, and generally carried the issues of clinical ethics front and center into the arena of complex, quaternary clinical care.

The history of clinical ethics has been weakest, however, in addressing the practical issues arising in the everyday clinical practice of medicine. The focus on ethics of quaternary medicine has led many clinicians to understand that ethical concerns are about unusual medicine and are best left to the experts, ethics committees, ethics consultants, and "ethicists." The conflict between moral obligations that may create a need for ethical analysis, however, is a profoundly common part of everyday clinical practice, identifiable in almost every clinician-patient encounter. If clinical ethics expertise is necessary in complex care, it is equally necessary in everyday clinical practice. Unlike the quaternary-care, extreme-case setting, where ethicists and ethics committees are accessible and legal consultation may be required, management of ethics issues in everyday clinical practice generally relies on the expertise and capacity for reasoning of the clinician and the team caring for the patient.

Pediatr Clin N Am 71 (2024) xiii–xvi
https://doi.org/10.1016/j.pcl.2023.09.003
0031-3955/24/© 2023 Published by Elsevier Inc.

While challenging, this is an idea worth celebrating because it brings attention to the routine clinician-patient encounter and can serve to remind the clinician of the importance of attending to the values that underlie patient care. Those values, no less influential for being so often unspoken, drive beliefs about the goals of care, the expectations about the clinician-patient relationship, the ideas of well-being and harm, and the identification of a satisfactory outcome, for both the clinician and the patient. In the setting of pediatric care, the essential triad of patient, parent, and clinician adds an extra dimension to the values of environment and requires additional expertise in navigation.

Medical ethics is a formal part of the curriculum in medical schools in North America. Most clinicians express awareness of the importance of clinical ethics. However, confidence about identifying and managing ethical concerns that impact routine patient care remains highly variable among clinicians. This issue of *Pediatric Clinics of North America* seeks to assist clinicians in identifying and managing ethical issues in the everyday practice of pediatrics.

Its focus is on the practical—a "how-to" approach to common concerns in pediatric care that arise out of conflicting values and moral obligations, using everyday cases to highlight and reinforce ideas.

Dr Mark Hughes presents some common frameworks for ethics and highlights one step-by-step approach that works well within the clinical arena, as it parallels the process of diagnostic decision making. This framework also works especially well as an outline for a team discussion of an ethics concern. Dr Lainie Ross offers an excellent analysis of one of the essential problems in pediatric medicine, understanding the duties and rights of parents in deciding for children. Drs Douglas Opel and Kimberly Sawyer present a very useful stepwise technique for shared decision making that can help bring values conflicts to light so they can be addressed and resolved. Dr Nicholas Jabre adds some insight into the impact of uncertainty on decision making, both for clinicians and for patients.

Moving to the more specific arenas of everyday ethics concerns in the pediatric setting, Dr Joseph Carrese's article uses the step-by-step framework presented by Dr Hughes and develops it specifically for the setting of outpatient pediatrics, using cases drawn from our own Johns Hopkins Harriet Lane Primary Care Clinic experience. Drs Renee Boss and Carrie Henderson bring focus to the expanding domain of pediatric medical complexity and present a rich discussion of managing disagreements around goals of care in the setting of complexity. Dr Rebecca Seltzer and Ms Simone Thompson highlight the particular anxieties confronted when identifying and responding to concerns about potential medical neglect and the involvement of outside agencies and authorities in the clinician-patient-family interaction. Dr Mary Ott, writing about the problem of confidentiality in the care of adolescent and young adult patients, offers ideas to give clinicians confidence in working with adolescents and their families. Finally, Drs Micah Hester and Skye Miner bring concerns about consent and assent into focus and recognize that the research context often overlaps with the clinical context in modern pediatrics. As a set, these articles offer a rich and well-rounded perspective on ethics in everyday clinical pediatrics and a valuable collection of tools with which to engage, analyze, and resolve commonplace but perplexing dilemmas.

A note of caution about autonomy in pediatric ethics. As you explore these excellent articles, please think carefully about the language of autonomy in clinical ethics. The duty to respect the autonomy of patients has a strong grip on the sensibilities of most clinicians trained in western medicine. Autonomy, understood as the capacity for self-rule, is fundamental to the experience of being human. The ability to develop a sense of the good specific to one's own goals and beliefs and the ability to act to promote that sense of the good are essential to human nature. To the extent that a person has that capacity, we respect their ability to do so, within important boundaries. In the clinical setting, this translates to the duty to respect a patient's rational decision to opt out of beneficial care, even though the clinician disagrees with the decision, even with the rationale. The conflict between the duty to promote well-being and the duty to respect the autonomy of a competent patient making bad choices is all too familiar to clinicians from every field of medicine.

The duty to respect the autonomy of a competent patient, however, does not transfer very easily to the pediatric setting, when the patient does not have capacity for decision making. One of the joys of pediatric practice is observing the development of autonomy as children grow to adolescents and then young adults. A primary goal of pediatrics is to protect, promote, and support the development of capacity and autonomy from the prenatal period to full adulthood. In the absence of fully developed capacity for decision making and in the setting of legal minority, we anticipate that parents are the most appropriate decision makers for their children. We honor parents as decision makers for their minor children because we presume that parents are best placed, by virtue of their love for and knowledge of the child, to make decisions that promote the child's general well-being. In addition, we honor parents as decision makers because they are morally and legally responsible for the well-being of their children and must manage the impact of medical choices on the child and the family. Finally, we have a societal belief in cohesive families as essential to a strong community, and honoring the parental role conforms to that belief. The language of respect for autonomy, however, does not fit here as a justification for parental authority as decision maker. In fact, the presumption that parents' wishes must be honored because clinicians have the duty to respect the parents' autonomy is dangerous and contrary to the duty of the pediatrician.

The duty to respect autonomy arises from the capacity for self-rule, the capacity to identify and act on an internal, personal sense of the good. Parents who are competent adults are free to make decisions for themselves that, while promoting that internal sense of the good, are potentially harmful. Parents are not equally free to make decisions for their children that, while promoting a parents' sense of the good, are likely to be harmful to the child.

Establishing the boundary between the fairly wide latitude we give competent adults in their role as parents to decide about their childs' medical care and the duty to step in to protect a child from bad decisions made by a competent adult is a primary challenge in clinical pediatrics. When is a choice about medical care bad enough to justify intervention, and how do we manage the collateral effects of intervening? Several of the articles that follow address facets of this issue and offer insight into the justifications, nuances, and sensitivities of challenging parental authority. The first step, however, is to be alert to the slippery application of the language of respect for parental autonomy to the parent-child-clinician interaction. With regard to respect for autonomy, the duty of a pediatric clinician is to honor parents in their role as family decision makers and work closely with them to support, protect, and promote the developing autonomy of the child.

CONFLICT OF INTEREST/DISCLOSURES

The guest editor has nothing to disclose.

Margaret R. Moon, MD, MPH
Department of Pediatrics
Johns Hopkins School of Medicine
Johns Hopkins Children's Center
1800 Orleans, Room 8491, Johns Hopkins
Baltimore, MD 21287, USA

E-mail address:
mmoon4@jhmi.edu

The Imperative of Ethics in Everyday Clinical Pediatrics

Margaret R. Moon, MD, MPH

KEYWORDS

• Ethics • Everyday • Clinical • Pediatrics • Values • Integrity

KEY POINTS

- Ethics is a method to balance competing values in everyday clinical practice.
- Competence in clinical ethics is crucial to competence in pediatrics.
- Clinicians should be able to identify and communicate the values that influence patient care decisions.

INTRODUCTION

Clinical ethics is necessary because medicine, especially pediatric medicine, necessarily involves values. At the heart of every clinician/patient/family encounter is an interaction around values, the values that inform our sense of health and well-being, harm, and suffering. Patients seek care to enhance well-being and avoid the harms of illness and suffering. Clinicians seek to promote well-being and minimize harms for the patient and the family. In pediatric care, the values that parents ascribe to parenting and family are also very much part of the interaction, as are the values that determine the clinician's approach to pediatric patients and their families. Because the goals of care themselves, well-being, harm avoidance, and relief from suffering entail concepts that are essentially value laden, competence in medicine requires the ability, and willingness to identify and respond to the effect of values on the clinical interaction.

The values that affect the clinical experience for both clinician and patient arise from a myriad of sources: religious, moral, professional, social, and cultural. Deeply held values have the power to create duties and impose limits. Values can color interpretation of facts and experience. Whenever values are involved in decision-making, as in every experience between clinicians and patients, there is opportunity for conflict related to values and their associated duties. Values-related conflicts are especially

Department of Pediatrics, Johns Hopkins University, School of Medicine, Johns Hopkins University, Berman Institute of Bioethics, 1800 Orleans Street, Room 8419, Baltimore, MD 2187, USA
E-mail address: mmoon4@jhu.edu

Pediatr Clin N Am 71 (2024) 1–8
https://doi.org/10.1016/j.pcl.2023.09.001
0031-3955/24/© 2023 Elsevier Inc. All rights reserved.

difficult when values are unspoken and presumptions about shared values remain unexplored and unchallenged.

Ethics is a method for analyzing conflicts between value-driven duties and obligations. Clinical ethics anticipates that conflicts are inevitable in the clinical setting and functions to explore and clarify conflicting duties and obligations with the goal to identify the action or set of possible actions that provides optimal balance between all the obligations that affect decisions about the plan of care.

"A worry about ethics typically emerges when serious political, scientific, and cultural changes are afoot."[1] The modern environment of health care—characterized by complexity, rapid changes in medical science, advancing technology, social and cultural discordance, and new patterns of information use and dissemination—highlights the importance of skill in managing values as part of the everyday clinical encounter.

As noted above, competence in medicine requires that practitioners develop sensitivity to ethical challenges raised by competing obligations, along with skills in addressing those challenges. This issue of Pediatric Clinics of North America focuses on clinical ethics issues that arise in every day pediatric practice and will offer practical guidance and case examples to help practitioners identify and begin to address commonplace conflicts between values and obligations in the clinical arena.

BACKGROUND: CLINICAL ETHICS IN THE CONTEXT OF BIOETHICS

Contextual grounding is needed to bring clinical ethics into focus. Clinical ethics is one dimension of bioethics. Within the larger framework of ethical philosophy, bioethics applies itself to the moral, legal, political, and social issues arising within the life sciences. Bioethics is the study of ethical issues arising in the life sciences at the intersections of health care, medical technology, and health and science policy. In its interdisciplinary nature, bioethics emphasizes that life science is a social activity. Life science, including medical science, is not just the creation and application of objective facts, but a cultural phenomenon influenced and informed by current social and political contexts. Bioethics is a field of study that analyzes the essential conflicts of interest in the life sciences. By most accounts, bioethics became an organized field of ethics in the mid-twentieth century, in response to rapid advances in medical technology that challenged our understanding of life, death, and what it is to be human.

In addition to clinical ethics, bioethics includes research ethics and public health or health policy ethics. Research ethics arose to navigate the protection of subjects of research. Research ethics highlights that research is so different from clinical care that the duties and obligations must be considered separately. Whereas clinical care is focused on the well-being of the patient, research uses subjects to produce generalizable knowledge to move medicine forward. The clinical relationship does not necessarily exist and so the primary duty of research ethics is to protect and respect the subject as a voluntary participant.

Public health ethics includes both the study of the principles that guide public health actions and the practice of applying public health policies to protect the health of communities. The distinction between public health ethics and clinical ethics is significant. Public health takes the health of communities as its focus, whereas clinical medicine focuses on the well-being of the individual patient. Conflicts naturally arise between the interests of the public and the interests of individual patients.[2]

Clinical ethics, then, is the only dimension of bioethics dedicated specifically to the practitioner–patient relationship and its essential goal of promoting the well-being of the individual patient. Much of the tradition of clinical ethics scholarship and practice has focused on complex, high-intensity, highly technical issues in tertiary or quaternary care, at the beginnings and ends of life. Conflicts in decisions about futility at the extremes of life, refusal or withdrawal of life-sustaining care, rationing rescue medicine, and justifiable risks in medical innovations are frequent case examples in the bioethics literature. This reflects the origins of modern clinical ethics as a field of study during the time when rapid advances in genetics, intensive care, and other technologies collided with new concerns about cost of care and human dignity. However, all of clinical medicine is value laden; clinical ethics is equally part of everyday clinical practice. When we restrict clinical ethics consideration to issues at the margins of life, we risk failing ourselves and our patients by neglecting the critically important challenges arising in our everyday work as clinicians.[3] "The ethics of the ordinary is just as much a part of health care ethics as the ethics of the extraordinary."[4]

CLINICAL ETHICS AND THE RISKS TO THE PROFESSION OF MEDICINE

A focus on clinical ethics as part of routine pediatric practice is particularly timely. The profession of medicine is at risk. A recent report from the Pew Research Center shows that among Americans age 18 to 49, fewer than 50% believe that doctors usually (1) care about patients' best interests, (2) do a good job with treatment recommendations, and (3) provide fair and accurate information. Even fewer have faith that doctors are transparent about conflicts of interest (15%) and admit mistakes and take responsibility (12%). Older Americans show more faith in medicine, but it is the 18 to 49 years age group that is most likely to have children requiring pediatric care.[5]

Although some of the loss of faith in medicine likely arises from current cultural phenomena such as the rise of anti-science dogma and identity politics that challenge scientific expertise, it is important for clinicians to realize that some of the current harm to the profession of medicine can be traced to failures to manage values conflicts effectively. Those harms are self-imposed but highly preventable. Expertise in clinical ethics is a practice in preventing the harms imposed by conflicts in values and their inherent obligations.

Failures of Integrity

The essential basis of an effective doctor–patient relationship is trust. Medicine works most effectively when the patient can trust that the doctor is working toward the patient's best interest and the doctor can trust that the patient is telling the truth. In the past decade, there have been heavily reported failures of trustworthiness in clinical medicine. Physicians overprescribing narcotics for financial gain and physicians sexually abusing vulnerable patients are some of the most sickening examples. The potential conflicts created by fee-for-service medicine, where unscrupulous practitioners can benefit financially by providing unnecessary care or by restricting access to necessary care cast a pall over the ideal doctor–patient relationship. Even conscientious physicians are faced with limiting optimal care to some patients due to insurance regulations and limits while providing that care to other better-insured patients. Prominent failures of integrity among high-profile leaders in medicine further erode confidence in the profession of medicine. The report that the chief medical officer of a highly regarded cancer institute resigned amid revelations that he failed to report millions of dollars of payments from drug companies and financial startups was highly publicized in popular media outlets.[6] Finally, the influence of outside interests on physicians has become so concerning to the public that the "Sunshine Act," which became law in 2010, requires that the pharmaceutical and medical technology industries publicly report payments to physicians.[7] Modern clinical medicine offers many reasons for our patients to question whether that basic tenet of the doctor–patient relationship that the doctor seeks the well-being of the patient over other interests is true. Natural suspicion about medicine and goals of the clinician increases the imperative to anticipate concerns, consider the impact of values conflicts, and develop skills in managing ethical issues in everyday practice.

Conflicts About the Goals of Medicine

Although prominent failures of integrity within the profession of medicine are a key influence on loss of faith in medicine, another is differences in understanding of the goals of medicine itself. Misalignment in perceptions of the goals of medicine can underlie conflicts within the profession as well as between physicians and patients. Consensus about the goals of medicine could help establish what patients should be able to expect from physicians, which dimensions of care are necessary and which are beyond the boundaries of a physician's duty, what health care delivery should seek to achieve, how to allocate scarce medical resources, which medical research should be funded, and how medical education should be focused.

Interestingly, there is only moderate current discussion of the goals of medicine as relevant to current practice. The latter part of the twentieth century saw the most recent broad debates about the goals of medicine. Howard Brody, a prominent philosopher of medicine, emphasized the importance of identifying goals of medicine, noting that medicine in not a neutral technique, but "a professional practice governed by a moral framework consisting of goals proper to medicine, role-specific duties, and clinical virtues. We call this framework "the internal morality of medicine." The professional integrity of physicians is constituted by loyalty and adherence to this internal morality."[8] Edmund Pellegrino and David Thomasma[9] argued for a narrow definition of the goals based on an understanding that medicine exists only because illness exists. The goals of medicine then are to heal illness, to return the body to its normal physiologic state.[10] Daniel Callahan and the Hastings Center developed a broader view, arguing that the rapid advances in medical technology and disease prevention challenged the narrow view of the meaning of medicine.[11] In the decades since Pellegrino, Callahan and Brody[12] highlighted the importance of the goals of medicine to set the internal morality and external boundaries of medicine, there has been remarkably little development of these ideas. As medical and health services technology continues to advance rapidly, it will be increasingly important to identify at least the boundaries of medicine, even if broad consensus on the goals is not available.

Three prominent approaches to the goals of medicine (**Table 1**) include what I will call here the hardline approach presented by the work of Edmund Pellegrino and David Thomasma,[9] the middle ground approach published by the Hastings Center[10] and the expansive approach based on the definition of health in the World Health Organization's constitution.[13]

The differences between these three theoretic constructions of the goals of medicine have very practical implications. Consider, for example, a healthy 17-year-old patient seeking rhinoplasty for cosmetic reasons. The patient has no respiratory or sinus-related concerns but is embarrassed by the size and contour of their nose. There is no indication of depression or diagnosed social anxiety disorder, but the patient is uncomfortable with their appearance and feels that life would be better if their nose were different. Per the hardline construction, it would be difficult to identify a disease state that could warrant the use of medical resources and biomedical technology. Consequently, the provider could say this was outside of the bounds of the profession and the health care system would be likely to deny the request.

Table 1 Approaches to the goals of medicine		
Hardline Approach	**Middle Ground Approach**	**Expansive Approach**
• Health is freedom from disease. • Goal of medicine is to promote health. • The primary use of biomedical technology is to treat physical or mental disease.	Goals of medicine are: • Prevention of disease, promotion of health • Relief of pain and suffering caused by maladies • Care and cure of maladies with a return to normal range of opportunity • Avoidance of early death and pursuit of a peaceful death	• Health is physical, mental, *and* social well-being. • *Goal* of medicine is to promote and protect *all* dimensions.

The middle ground construction, using the very broad term "malady" could identify unhappiness with one's appearance as a malady. Or perhaps note that in our society, with its narrow range of perceptions of beauty, having an unusually prominent nose can limit opportunity. In that case, the provider might be more likely to approve the request as within the bounds of the profession and the health care system would be less likely to deny the request.

The expansive construction would identify feeling ugly as having negative impact on mental and social well-being. Within that construction, approval of cosmetic rhinoplasty would be solidly within the expectations a patient would have of a physician and a health care system.

Cosmetic surgery is so common in current practice that this case seems to make a moot point. If the clinical situation is more complex, the issue becomes better defined. Imagine the same healthy 17 year old. Instead of rhinoplasty in the absence of a dysfunctional nasal system, the patient would like to have their legs removed below the knee and replaced by a set of the recently developed and amazing new prosthetic legs that would allow them to run longer without progressive pain from overuse. The patient is a competitive runner and has a family history of osteoarthritis. The patient believes sincerely that running is his source of social and emotional well-being.

Although this case is purposefully absurd, the point is that differences in beliefs about the goals of medicine can easily create conflict about the duties of the physician to the patient and the justifiable limits on the use of health care resources. The hardline construction would reject the idea that there is any current disease state and have an easy time rejecting this as inconsistent with the goals of medicine and out of the bounds of the profession. The middle ground construction, though, might struggle. The prevention of osteoarthritis and its consequent limited opportunity to find joy in running might be argued here. The expansive construction seems to justify boundless expectations of the role of the physician in responding to a patient's sense of well-being. The relevant question would be whether the heartfelt desire to continue competitive running a dimension of health that could prompt a duty from the practitioner.

In the absence of broad professional consensus about the goals of medicine, individual practitioners should work to clarify their own beliefs about the goals of medicine and how those goals set boundaries around the obligations of the profession. If the conclusion sets a practitioner apart from others in the profession, or even in their own practice group, further reflection might be needed. Once a clinician's beliefs

Table 2
Public health ethics and clinical ethics comparison

Public Health Ethics Framework	Clinical Ethics Framework
Primary relationship is to the community.	Primary relationship is the practitioner–patient.
Goal is maximal well-being of the community.	Goal is to promote the well-being of the individual patient.
The "good" is socially defined.	The "good" is defined by the individual patient.
Policy and practice emphasize community benefits.	Practice is individualized and patient-centered.
Social justice can take precedence over individual autonomy.	Respect for individual autonomy is a central tenet.
Uniform and compulsory measures are accepted if indicated for community benefit.	Compulsion and coercion are to be avoided.

are reasonably settled, the challenge is to be consistent and transparent in applying those beliefs in their own practice. Many simple conflicts in everyday clinical practice can be avoided if the patient what to expect from the practitioner and the values that set those expectations. Consider this preventive ethics for medical practice.

Conflicts Between Public Health and Clinical Ethics

A more recent risk to the trust basis of the practitioner–patient relationship is aligned with the growth of public health as a field of study and practice. Many practitioners, especially physicians, have studied public health as part of medical training. Commitment to the goals of public health, including promoting the health of communities, addressing the problem of over expenditure on health care, emphasizing disease prevention, and promoting social justice in health care is part of widely understood to be among the goals of the medical professions. The challenge is that the focus of public health is very different from the focus of clinical care. The focus of public health is the well-being of communities. The focus of clinical care, of the practitioner–patient relationship, is well-being of the individual patient. As summarized in **Table 2** below, public health ethics and clinical ethics naturally conflict.

Public health is a tremendously important practice. Many of the most valuable advances in life expectancy and overall health in the twentieth century came about as a result of public health science and practice. Consider vaccination, family planning, motor vehicle safety, safer and healthier foods, recognition of tobacco as a hazard, and decline in deaths from coronary artery disease.[14] These are just some of the incredible benefits of a robust focus on public health science and practice.

The risk to the profession of medicine comes when an individual wears both the public health practitioner hat and the clinical medicine practitioner hat at the same time. If patients sense that recommendations are promoting an outcome other than their individual well-being, they have reason to wonder which set of goals and which ethical framework is driving recommendations. Common examples might be a recommendation to use a cheaper drug instead of the fancy, highly advertised drug a patient has requested, or particularly in pediatric practice, a decision to end a clinical relationship with a family who has become vaccine hesitant. The basis of the effective practitioner–patient relationship is trust that the practitioner seeks the patient's well-being above other goals. Practitioners must work to promote both public health goals and the unique patient's well-being. Patients should, however, be included in understanding which values are driving the practitioner's decision-making within an encounter.

SUMMARY

The self-imposed risks to the profession of medicine are profound. As medical professionals, we have a duty to promote and protect the integrity of medical science and to help our patients maintain a rational faith in our practice. As a profession, we must demand integrity of ourselves and our systems. We should seek to attend more carefully to the values that underly our individual practice and our professional identities, including values related to the goals of medicine and beliefs about the balance between duties to the public's health and duties to the patient within the clinician/patient relationship. As clinicians, one of our best tools is a robust and consistent use of clinical ethics to guide decision-making when values conflicts arise.

As ethicist Peter Singer noted "Every clinician knows that bioethics is important. What is often missing is how to best approach bioethics problems in a practical way."[15] The articles that follow will help all pediatric practitioners develop a practical approach to problems in everyday clinical ethics.

DISCLOSURES

No disclosures to report.

REFERENCES

1. Callahan D. Bioethics and Policy – a history. The Hastings Center Bioethics Briefings. 2015. Available at: https://www.thehastingscenter.org/briefingbook/bioethics-and-policy-a-history/. Accessed February 22, 2023.
2. CDC Office of Science. "Public Health Ethics". Available at: https://www.cdc.gov/os/integrity/phethics/index.htm. Accessed March 17, 2023.
3. Komesaroff P. From bioethics to microethics: Ethical debate and clinical medicine. In: Komesaroff P, editor. Troubled bodies: critical perspectives on postmodernism, medical ethics, and the body. Durham, NC: Duke University Press; 1995. p. 62–86.
4. Caplan Al. The morality of the mundane. In: Kane RA, Caplan AL, editors. Everyday ethics: resolving dilemmas in nursing home life. New York: Springer; 1990. p. pp37–50.
5. Funk C et al. Pew research center august 2, 2019 "trust and mistrust in american's views of scientific experts" pp 27-34. Available at: https://www.pewresearch.org/science/2019/08/02/americans-generally-view-medical-professionals-favorably-but-about-half-consider-misconduct-a-big-problem/. Accessed November 14, 2022.
6. Ornstein C and Thomas K. Top cancer researcher fails to disclose corporate financial ties in major research journals. Available at: https://www.nytimes.com/2018/09/08/health/jose-baselga-cancer-memorial-sloan-kettering.html. Accessed February 20 2023.
7. 111th Congress of the United States. S.301 - Physician payments sunshine act of 2009. Available at: https://www.congress.gov/bill/111th-congress/senate-bill/301/text. Accessed March 10 2023.

8. Miller F, Brody H. Cosmetic surgery and the internal morality of medicine. Camb Q Healthc Ethics 2000;9:353–64.

9. Thomasma DC, Pellegrino ED. Philosophy of medicine as the source for medical ethics. Metamedicine 1981;2:5–11.

10. Pellegrino E. The internal morality of clinical medicine: a paradigm for the ethics of the helping and healing professions. J Med Philos 2001;26:559–79.

11. Callahan D. The goals of medicine. setting new priorities. Hastings Cent Rep 1996;26:S1–27.

12. Brody H. The physician-patient relationship: Models and criticisms. Theor Med Bioeth 1987;8:205–20.

13. World Health Organization. Constitution of the World Health Organization. Available at: https://www.who.int/about/governance/constitution. Accessed January 17, 2023.

14. CDC Morbidity and Mortality Review. ten great public health achievements, United States 1900-1999. Available at: https://www.cdc.gov/mmwr/preview/mmwrhtml/00056796.htm. Accessed April 2, 2023.

15. Singer P. Introduction. In: Singer P, Viens A, editors. Cambridge textbook of of bioethics. 1st edition. Cambridge: Cambridge University Press; 2003. p. 5.

How to "Do Ethics" in Pediatrics Practice
A Framework for Addressing Everyday Ethics Issues

Mark T. Hughes, MD, MA[a,b],*

KEYWORDS

• Ethics • Morality • Virtues • Principles • Professional obligations • Decision making

KEY POINTS

Stepwise approach to evaluating a clinical ethics concern.

- When a clinical case bothers a pediatrician, the first step is to explain why the case is concerning.
- To define a moral problem, the pediatrician should identify the rule, principle, virtue, obligation, or value that is at stake.
- A useful systematic framework can ensure all morally salient features have been considered by organizing the facts of the case in terms of medical condition, patient and parent perspective, and contextual features.
- The pediatrician should determine how much the minor patient can participate in the decision-making process.
- After finding guidance from various ethics sources, the pediatrician should deliberate about the options and decide on a morally defensible course of action.

INTRODUCTION

"Doing ethics" in clinical medicine is all about problem-solving. The pediatrician has to understand the circumstances of a particular case and come up with a plan that is ethically sound. The solution has to comport with the goals of the therapeutic alliance with the patient and their parent(s) or caregivers.[1,2] The course of action chosen must also be in line with the values, principles, and virtues of their profession. To accomplish this, the clinician needs a systematic process for gathering, organizing, and analyzing the facts of a case in light of its morally salient features. This article presents a

[a] Department of Medicine, Johns Hopkins University School of Medicine; [b] Berman Institute of Bioethics
* General Internal Medicine, 601 N. Caroline Street, JHOC Room 7143, Baltimore, MD 21287-0941.
E-mail address: mhughes2@jhmi.edu

Pediatr Clin N Am 71 (2024) 9–26
https://doi.org/10.1016/j.pcl.2023.09.002
0031-3955/24/© 2023 Elsevier Inc. All rights reserved.

Box 1

Stepwise approach for addressing ethics issues

1. What is the provider's concern? Why does this case bother the provider?

2. Is this ethics? Does the concern arise from a conflict between moral obligations, values, or virtues?

3. Who are the stakeholders?
   A. Who are the moral agents?
   B. Who are the informants to identify the facts and define relevant values and duties?
   C. What personal/professional experiences inform the provider's approach to this case?

4. What are the facts of the case? Is additional information needed?
   A. Medical Condition:
      1. What are the physical, mental, and/or social deficits with or without treatment?
      2. What are the indications and goals of treatment?
      3. What is the recommended treatment and its benefits and risks of harm?
      4. What are the alternative treatments and their benefits and risks of harm?
      5. What are the probabilities of success, prognosis, and uncertainties of treatment?
   B. Patient/Parent Perspective
      1. How much can the child participate in decision making?
      2. Is the condition one for which the child can make their own decisions?
      3. Does the minor have decision making capacity?
      4. Does the parent or guardian have decision making capacity?
      5. What are the treatment preferences of the patient and/or parent/guardian?
      6. What are the goals of care for the patient and/or parent/guardian, including any quality of life considerations?
   C. Contextual Features
      1. Is there a need to protect the patient's confidentiality from the parent/guardian?
      2. What familial, cultural, or religious issues might influence treatment decisions?
      3. Are financial or insurance concerns affecting treatment decisions?
      4. Are there concerns for child neglect or abuse?
      5. Are the decisions of the parent challengeable?
      6. Are legal considerations affecting any of the stakeholders?
      7. What professional or institutional factors are influencing the provider's perspective?
      8. Does the provider have any conflicts of interest or conflicts of obligation?

5. Are there other sources of information to provide guidance in helping to resolve the issue?
   A. Paradigm cases or case law
   B. Professional guidelines
   C. Helpful literature on this ethics issue
   D. Other lenses through which to look at case: Ethic of care, Narrative ethics

6. What are the possible options and what action will be taken?
   A. What choices are *possible*? What are their tradeoffs (advantages and disadvantages)?
   B. What *should* be done? Does clinical ethical reasoning justify one choice as preferable?
   C. What *will* be done? Do impediments limit the choices of what can be done?

7. Once an action is taken, what are the consequences? Does the outcome require a re-evaluation of the plan?

---

framework for performing an ethics case analysis (**Box 1**). To illustrate how the stepwise approach works, the following case is commented on at each step.

CASE

Patient Jane is a 13-year-old girl with mild intellectual developmental disability who is being seen for a well child visit at the beginning of the school year. Her evaluation reveals her to be a healthy teenager who is excited to be going back to school. She had menarche at age 12 and is developing secondary sexual characteristics. Her 29-year-old mother Mary requests the patient be prescribed oral contraceptive pills (OCP), because she has seen boys in the neighborhood noticing her daughter. She worries what could happen to her daughter going to and from school or when she is out in the neighborhood. Her mother does not want to disclose what type of medication the OCP is or what it is for. She plans to tell Jane that the OCP is a vitamin. Mary is adamant that her child not be informed. There is a decision to be faced: whether to prescribe the OCP in the first place, and if prescribed, whether to honor the mother's demand not to disclose the indication for the medication. Consultation with colleagues in the group practice elicits different opinions on what to do. Some say that this is lying and lying is never acceptable. Some say it is harm reduction and acceptable. Some say they feel legally required to follow the mother's wishes as she is responsible for the child's well-being. What course of action should be taken?

CASE EVALUATION STEP 1
What Is Your Concern? Why Does This Case Bother You?

When a clinical case or situation is bothering a pediatrician, the first step is to define why it is a concern and whether a review from the ethics perspective is warranted. Often, a triggering event for the clinician in a case will activate an emotional reaction (eg, anxiety, anger, guilt, sadness).[3] Empathic arousal can provide a clue that something of ethical importance is at stake. It may be that seeing the suffering of the patient or family moves the clinician to compassion.[4] It may be that the uncertainty of a situation or how it will unfold causes anxiety. It may be that the clinician's own limitations in knowledge on how best to proceed are the concern. It may be that there has been a communication failure along the way, and the therapeutic relationship is affected. While all of these concerns have ethical underpinnings in light of the internal morality of medicine,[5] they might be answered or addressed without reliance on an ethical framework. Ethics comes into play when a moral principle, value, or obligation is being challenged.

It helps for the clinician to articulate the concern to determine if a moral principle or value is being challenged. Moral sensitivity is the first step in recognizing a moral issue is involved in a situation. It entails that the pediatrician sees themselves as a moral agent and that their actions have consequences for other people.[6,7] Through socialization into medicine, the pediatrician appreciates the norms of the profession.[8] By stating the problem clearly, the pediatrician discovers what their role is in determining what course of action to take and how they, the patient, and others involved in the situation will be affected. Answering the first question also provides the scope of additional information or insight needed to reach a resolution to the concern.

Step 1 Finding: Statement of Specific Concern
Concern: "The mother of my 13-year-old patient wants me to prescribe an oral contraceptive and not tell the patient what it is for."

CASE EVALUATION STEP 2
Is This Ethics? Does the Concern Arise from a Conflict Between Moral Obligations, Values, or Virtues?

Various approaches to ethical analysis are possible (**Table 1**). For the clinician, it is helpful to have a simple, familiar approach to define the moral problem. A philosopher or ethicist may delve deeper into ethical inquiry, but for everyday ethics issues, the pediatrician can start with a basic framework. One could rely on common morality, using ordinary moral experience and applying it to particular contexts, such as the

Table 1
Approaches to ethics

Common Morality[a]

General moral rules:
1. Do not kill.
2. Do not cause pain.
3. Do not disable.
4. Do not deprive of freedom.
5. Do not deprive of pleasure.
6. Do not deceive.
7. Keep your promises.
8. Do not cheat.
9. Obey the law.
10. Do your duty.

Charter on Professionalism

Fundamental Principles:
1. *Primacy of patient welfare*: Serving the patient's best interests; establishing trust
2. *Patient autonomy*: Being honest; empowering the patient to make informed decisions
3. *Social justice*: Promoting fair distribution of resources; eliminating discrimination
   Professional Responsibilities/Commitments:
   1. Professional competence in knowledge/skills
   2. Honesty with patients
   3. Patient confidentiality
   4. Maintain appropriate relations with patients
   5. Improve quality of care
   6. Improve access to equitable health care
   7. Just distribution of finite resources
   8. Use and integrity of scientific knowledge
   9. Manage conflicts of interest
   10. Responsibilities to set standards

Virtues in Medical Practice

Fidelity to trust and promise:	Inviting and upholding the patient's trust in the relationship
Benevolence:	Intending every act to be in the patient's interest
Effacement of self-interest:	Preventing exploitation of the patient
Compassion and caring:	Feeling something of the patient's experience of illness
Fortitude	Committing to a moral good through sustained courage
Intellectual honesty:	Acknowledging ignorance and being humble to admit it
Justice:	Adjusting what is owed to the specific needs of the patient
Prudence:	Possessing practical wisdom; deliberation and discernment

The Four Principles

Respect for Autonomy:	Respecting and supporting autonomous decisions
Nonmaleficence:	Avoiding the causation of harm
Beneficence:	Relieving, lessening, or preventing harm; providing benefits; balancing benefits against risks and costs
Justice	Fairly distributing benefits, risks, and costs

[a] Rules have to be to applied and interpreted in the professional context.

profession of medicine. For instance, Clouser remarks that the general moral rule of not infringing on freedom leads to the particular professional obligation of obtaining informed consent.[9] Common morality has some appeal because it provides a detailed procedure for dealing with conflicts.[10] The challenge would be applying the rules and ideals of common morality to the medical context. A second approach would be to invoke professional responsibilities commonly known to physicians, such as those articulated in the Physician Charter on professionalism. The Charter, which is endorsed by the American Academy of Pediatrics (AAP), starts with 3 core principles: primacy of patient welfare, patient autonomy, and social justice.[11] Another option for ethical analysis (and which can be linked to professionalism) would be reference to virtue theory—namely the virtues the pediatrician is striving to uphold in their moral character as a physician.[12,13] A fourth option would be the 4 principles articulated by Beauchamp and Childress.[14] The principles are widely known in contemporary medicine and therefore create a useful starting point.

After stating the problem or concern, the next step is to name the ethical obligations or values involved. Moral intuition directs the pediatrician to recognize something is wrong, but it would be helpful to identify specific role obligations involved.[15] Naming which of the 4 principles is at stake (and how) can be a starting point—all 4 are often involved. For difficult cases, 2 or more principles are typically in conflict. The nature of a moral dilemma is that one obligation directs the pediatrician to act one way, but another obligation leads them to act in a different way, such that both obligations cannot be fulfilled. It can also be the case that fulfilling a professional obligation may impact a virtue that the pediatrician is trying to uphold. This step is generally assessed from the perspective of the clinician and the responsibilities, virtues, or values they are trying to uphold in service to the patient. Nonetheless, it is important not to lose sight of the patient's or family's perspective and what values or goals they are hoping to achieve.

Step 2 Finding: Conflicting Moral Obligations
Among the 4 principles, respect for autonomy manifests both in respecting the mother's decision-making as a parent on behalf of her daughter but also respect for Jane's burgeoning autonomy as a teenager. Although Jane is a minor and has cognitive disability, she is at an age when she can be making certain decisions about her body, her health, and her life. Depending on her level of understanding, she may be able to assent to taking a medication, which entails that she knows what the medication is for. From the Charter on Professionalism, empowering patients to make their own decisions requires being honest with them. Beneficence is also a factor in the case—it would be in her best interest to avoid an unwanted pregnancy, but taking an oral contraceptive comes with the burden of taking a daily pill and having awareness of potential side effects and drug interaction. Nonmaleficence comes in the form of causing dignitary harm to the patient by lying to her if her mother's wishes are to be followed. If Jane later finds out that her pediatrician was dishonest, she may lose trust in the provider and in health care. The virtue of fidelity to trust and fulfilling the inherent promise of the therapeutic relationship is potentially jeopardized. Other virtues at stake are benevolence, compassion and caring, and ultimately prudence in figuring out what the right thing to do is in this situation.

CASE EVALUATION STEP 3
Who are the Stakeholders?

A stakeholder is a person, group, or organization who has an interest in the health care decision or action. Given the negative historical connotations associated with stakeholder, "interested parties" may be a more appropriate term.[16] Because the stakes can be high in ethical decision-making, the term "stakeholder" will be used in the stepwise approach. The stakeholders will include the moral agents involved in the decision or action. To qualify as a moral agent, an individual must have motives that can be judged by others in the moral realm and the individual must be able to make moral judgments about the rightness and wrongness of their actions.[17] In the therapeutic pediatric relationship, the physician and the decision maker (a parent or sometimes a patient if they are capable of autonomous decisions) have moral status due to their moral agency. The moral agents will clearly be informants to define the relevant values and duties at stake, but informants can include other members of the interdisciplinary team, other family members or friends, and representatives of organizations ranging from child protective services to institutional administrators. Good ethics starts with good facts, so it is important to cast as broad a net as necessary to gather information that will be relevant to a case. Part of that fact-gathering is self-reflection by the provider to understand how past experiences influence their own approach to a case. These could be personal experiences of dealing with illness in oneself or one's family, or they could be professional experiences of similar cases that went well or poorly based on decisions made. Self-reflection is also an opportunity to check oneself for implicit biases.[18]

Step 3 Finding: The stakeholders
The main stakeholders in the case are the physician, the patient Jane, and her mother Mary. It needs to be determined if Jane's father is involved in her life and has a role in decision making. Other potential moral agents include family members (e.g., grandparents, aunts, uncles) who might be involved in her upbringing and hence might be asked to be complicit in lying about the intent of the OCP. Similarly, other members of the health care team may be involved in clarifying her medication list. Informants could include nurses or social workers who have interacted with Jane and her mother, or potentially teachers or school officials who might know more about Jane's school or home environment. The physician can ask themselves what past experiences have shaped their attitudes about adolescent sexuality, patients with intellectual disability, personal values around truthtelling, and other issues triggered by the case.

CASE EVALUATION STEP 4
Organizing the Facts: What Are the Facts of the Case? Is Additional Information Needed?

The fourth step in the framework is to organize the information that is known and to determine what additional information would be helpful in proving justification for different paths of action. As seen in **Box 1**, the 3 categories are (a) Medical Condition, (b) Patient/Parent Perspective, and (c) Contextual Features. This is similar to the familiar and helpful 4 Topic method,[19] but puts Quality of Life questions under Medical Condition as the physical, mental, and/or social deficits that are expected from the condition or the treatment. The patient's or parent's subjective assessment of quality of life is also covered by the goals of care defined by the patient or parent in the Patient/Parent Perspective category.

Medical Condition
The Medical Condition category pertains primarily to the principles of beneficence and non-maleficence. Pediatricians will be comfortable with the questions pertaining to Medical Condition, as they will be consonant with their role in diagnosing, treating, and educating. Often in pediatrics, the condition will not be a disease or illness but instead how to keep the child healthy and prevent diseases in the future (eg, vaccination, healthy habits). Treatment decisions might also include the diagnostic tests needed to establish a diagnosis, and the burdens associated with the tests. The indications, benefits, and risks of the recommended treatment and alternatives should be

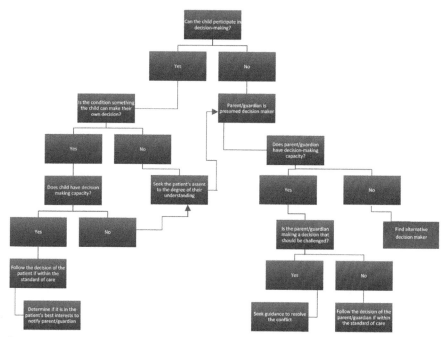

Fig. 1. Determination of who will participate in clinical decisions.

specified. Risks should be considered not only in terms of physical, psychological, or social harms but also any costs or burdens associated with adhering to the treatment. In reviewing the case, the pediatrician should be clear about the probabilities of success of the recommended treatment and how the alternatives compare. It is also possible that uncertainties will be part of the treatment assessment, especially if the patient has other comorbidities or the treatment has multiple steps. Lastly, the framework asks the pediatrician to specify the overall goals of treatment from the clinician's perspective.

Step 4(a) Finding: Medical Condition. The treatment under consideration is oral contraceptive pills. We do not know enough about the patient's condition to determine if this is warranted. More information is needed about the patient's sexual history. Her mother seems to be concerned that Jane could be at risk for being taken advantage of sexually in light of her cognitive disability. For another 13-year-old girl who is sexually active, an OCP could certainly be an option. Other forms of contraception could also be considered, with >90% effectiveness.[20] The patient would also have to be counseled on safer sexual practices and prevention of sexually transmitted diseases.

Step 4(b) Patient/Parent Perspective. The Patient/Parent Perspective category addresses the principle of respect for autonomy, which more accurately might be phrased as *respect for persons* for 2 reasons. First, the autonomy of the parent as decision maker is not absolute. Second, the pediatrician must still consider the perspective of the child even if the child does not have autonomy. An algorithm for who is involved in the decision-making process and how is shown in **Fig. 1**. The first question in Patient/Parent Perspective category addresses the extent to which the minor child can participate in the decision-making process. Infants and young children will obviously not be able to make decisions but can exhibit behaviors making them more or less receptive to the interventions being considered. As children get older, they will gain greater ability to participate in decisions and should be educated about what is happening with their bodies and the medical treatments being given to them. Some minors will have the legal right to make their own decisions if they are emancipated (in light of marriage, military service, or demonstration of being financially independent and living apart from their parents). In other cases, the adolescent might be deemed to be a Mature Minor.[21,22] Depending on the jurisdiction and the age of the patient, certain treatment decisions (eg, reproductive health) are permitted to be made by adolescents.[23] Generally, for this to occur, the pediatrician needs to determine that the adolescent has sufficient maturity and intelligence to understand and appreciate the benefits and risks of the treatment, as well as the long-term consequences. For confidential care in the delivery of certain treatments, the clinician has to be of the opinion that the treatment is necessary and for the minor's personal benefit, and that the patient has the ability to make a reasoned decision based on the knowledge the clinician has provided. For some adolescent health decisions regarding risky behaviors such as sexual activity or substance use, harm reduction techniques are employed to decrease the negative consequences of behaviors.[24]

The second question in the Patient/Parent Perspective category concerns whether the condition is one for which the minor patient can make their own decisions. If a minor patient is statutorily considered an adult or is legally permitted to make health care decisions in certain situations, the informed consent process entails that they are given sufficient medical information by which to make a decision. The Rule of Sevens is a shorthand method of determining age cutoffs for children to understand medical information.[25] It has been argued that adolescents over age 13 have the ability to understand medical information and express treatment preferences. A child's capacity for involvement in medical decision-making will be influenced by their prior experience in making different types of health decisions.[26] Neurocognitively, the integration of the socioemotional system (more impulsive and intuitive) and the cognitive-control system (more volitional and deliberate) typically does not occur until age greater than 20.[23] Adolescents may have a tendency toward risk-taking and to be influenced by emotion and external pressures. Settings characterized by "unhurried deliberation in the absence of emotional arousal" may allow a minor as young as age 16 to have the capacity to make medical decisions.[27] Acknowledging emotions and allowing more time for deliberation can aid in shared decision-making.[28]

If the pediatric patient is in a position to make their own decisions, the clinician should assess decision-making capacity. Decision-making capacity has 4 components—understanding, appreciation, reasoning ability, and making a decision.[29] If the child does not have decision-making capacity, they might still be able to provide assent.[30] Giving children without capacity a sense of control over some decisions shows them respect as persons.[31] When minors with or without capacity refuse treatment that is efficacious, the pediatrician may need to challenge their decision.[32] For minors capable of (and permitted to) making their own decision, the pediatrician may wish to discuss with the adolescent whether it would be in their best interests to involve their parents or guardians in the decision-making process. There may be situations in which the clinician judges that parental involvement would be prudent, and depending on the issue and the jurisdiction, the pediatrician may have the discretion to notify parents or guardians, even against the objection of the minor patient. Such a decision would have to be made carefully and with consideration of its effects on the therapeutic relationship with the adolescent.

In a large majority of cases, parents will be involved in making health care decisions for or with their child. One of the first items to sort out is whether this is 1 parent or 2 parents, and if 2 parents, whether they agree on the health care decisions for the child. The pediatrician should determine if the parent has decision-making capacity. Families in which the parent has impaired judgment as a result of substance use warrant special consideration. (Bondi) It may be advisable in those situations to defer nonurgent pediatric care until valid consent can be obtained from the parent or from another suitable authorized decision maker.[33] It may be necessary to pursue guardianship. The safety of the child would also be a consideration in such cases, and the clinician would have to make a clinical judgment about reporting to child protective services. Pediatricians may also encounter situations in which the caregiver accompanying the child to their medical care has an informal kinship relationship with the patient.[34] Jurisdictions will vary in terms of how much an informal kinship caregiver can make health care decisions for a child. Although the authorized decision maker for the child could potentially be a parent, guardian, or informal kinship caregiver, for the remainder of the article, we will focus on the parent as the decision maker.

If the parent has decision-making capacity, the next question in the Patient/Parent Perspective category asks what the decision maker's preferences are in regard to the recommended treatment and the alternative treatments. The parent integrates the information given by the physician with their family's values and needs to determine what they think is in the child's bests interests. The goals of care from the parent's perspective could be aimed toward maintaining the child's health, supporting their growth and development, or treating a particular disease. Goals might be focused on quality of life considerations, especially if a disease process is associated with high physical and/or psychological symptom burden. If the proposed treatment adversely affects quality of life, a parent's goals may lead them to refuse the treatment. Parents are granted some discretion in refusing recommended treatment. Parents exercise discretion in making a wide range of child-rearing decisions, including where they live, where they attend school, what religion they practice. Within the family construct, parents may have to weigh the interests of 1 child with the interests of their other children. Some medical decisions on behalf of their child will be made in light of the costs and burdens to the entire family. So there may be times when a parent's decision is not in the "best" interest of the patient, but it may be good enough.

Step 4(b) Finding. Not enough is known about Jane at this point. Although she has an intellectual disability, she may have the capacity to make decisions about contraception. More history needs to be obtained on whether she is sexually active or wants to be. The pediatrician needs to explore with Jane's mother how real the threat is of Jane's vulnerability to the boys in the neighborhood—is this an overly protective mother or have some events occurred that make her worried? Although Mary has stated the preference for not telling Jane about what the oral contraceptive pills are, she does not explain why. Is she concerned that introducing sexuality to Jane might lead her to become interested in it? Is Jane's mother not ready to see her daughter grow up? A fuller understanding of the mother's goals of care is needed before proceeding.

Step 4(c) Contextual Features. The Contextual Features category considers factors on both the patient's side and the physician's side that can influence care decisions. These features address the principle of justice, especially in terms of fairness in accounting for the background of the patient and family. The category also speaks to the process by which the pediatrician fulfills their societal role of protecting vulnerable persons in the community. The first question highlights an aspect of adolescent medicine in which the patient may be making treatment decisions without the involvement of the parent. The clinician needs to appreciate the contours of protecting the patient's confidentiality and whether or not it is advisable to notify the parent of the clinical issue at hand. Rationales have been advanced as to why it is important to provide confidential care to adolescents for issues such as reproductive and sexual health.[35] Depending on the treatment issues, jurisdictions vary as to how much parental notification is required and whether the pediatrician has discretion in making decisions about whether to breach confidentiality if they feel it is in the interests of the patient or a third party at risk of harm. A separate but related issue is whether the clinician has any obligation for mandatory reporting to governmental agencies (eg, public health reporting of sexually transmitted diseases). If the clinician feels that disclosure to the parent or guardian could pose harm to the adolescent, then this gives greater weight to protecting the confidential information.

The next issue to determine within contextual features is whether other information about who the patient is as a person has an impact on the care decisions being made. To some extent, this would be covered in the assessment of the medical condition. For adolescents, the HEEADSSS methods of interviewing will cover various aspects of the psychosocial review of systems. The mnemonic includes Home environment, Education and employment, Eating, peer-related Activities, Drugs, Sexuality, Suicide/depression, and Safety from injury and violence.[36] While HEEADSSS is primarily used for preventive health purposes, it provides an opportunity to learn about and address any social health inequities.[37] For the ethics case analysis, explicitly stating whether there are relevant familial, cultural, or religious factors in the exploration of the goals of care with the patient and/or parent or guardian is a good reminder to deliver patient-centered and family-centered care.[38] Familial issues include who else lives in the household, education level of authorized decision makers, health literacy, and whether other family members are dealing with health concerns. Cultural factors may be relevant if there are particular health or illness beliefs, behaviors, or rituals that are practiced within the culture. The family's primary language may affect their ability to understand medical information (and should prompt the inclusion of trained medical interpreters). Some families will rely heavily on their faith in making medical decisions.[39] It will be context dependent on how much to respect religious beliefs of parents when making health care decisions for a child—with the test being whether the life or health of the child is jeopardized by the parental decision (eg, lifesaving blood transfusion for a child raised in a Jehovah's Witness congregation; mandatory vaccination for a child in an orthodox Jewish family).

Financial issues should also be explored. The child's health insurance status and the family's ability to pay for the recommended treatment may influence parental decisions. With help from other members of the interdisciplinary team, such as social workers, it helps to clarify sources of income and employment status within the family (eg, how feasible is it for the parent or authorized decision maker to take time off from work to participate in the child's health care?). Financial matters may also influence the clinician's perspective. Does cost of a medication affect the range of options that are offered to the patient? Does the pediatrician worry about billing concerns or allocation of resources?

Another important contextual feature is whether there are any concerns for abuse or neglect of the child.[40] If abuse or neglect are suspected, reporting to child protective services in the interest of child safety takes high priority. If child protective services have already been involved in a child's case, then the health care team needs to determine whether the parents retain authority to make medical decisions for the child.

Next in the contextual features is whether the pediatrician has any concerns about medical neglect based on the parent's decision. If a parent refuses the recommended treatment, a threshold exists for when the pediatrician can contest a parent's decision. The harm principle can be invoked to challenge a parent's refusal of recommended treatment.[41] The harm principle holds that a parent's refusal can be questioned if it poses a risk of serious harm to the child—eg, not meeting the child's basic needs or causing significant morbidity. If this occurs, then the pediatrician should try to resolve the conflict by conducting more discussions with the parent to determine if the refusal is due to lack of understanding, irrational beliefs, or a mistake. It may be helpful to get a second opinion, involve an ethics committee, or compromise with the parent to lower the potential harm to the child down to an acceptable level.[42] A last resort would be to seek state involvement in the interests of the child. Some commentators have argued that the state could also intervene against a parent's interests in child-raising in the interests of communal and public health.[43,44]

Legal concerns may affect decision-making. A parent may be incarcerated or under the authority of law enforcement. Parents may be in a custody battle with each other, or divorce settlements have removed custodial rights of 1 parent. As mentioned earlier, a guardian may already have been appointed for the child in situations when both parents are not able to fulfill their parenting role. From the physician aspect, the pediatrician may be worried about future legal liability or already getting guidance from risk managers about actions to take. They may also need to take steps to prevent claims of abandonment if they decide to end the therapeutic relationship.[45]

Attributes of the physician or the institution where they practice can influence the decision-making process. It is possible that the institution is exerting pressure on the pediatrician overtly or subtly. The past few years have seen increasing recognition of the effects of implicit bias and structural racism on the delivery of care.[46] Institutional policies may dictate the range of options offered to patients. Quality metrics may influence the physician's practice behavior, such as what they recommend to patients. Other members of the clinical team could have opinions that differ from the pediatrician. If the physician is also a teacher, there may be conflicts of obligation with regard to their duty to the patient and their duty to the learner or trainee. Conflicts of obligation could also be seen with clinical investigators who have to follow clinical trial protocol when managing a patient. The physician also has to attend to their obligations to their family. Lastly, the physician may be swayed by conflicts of interest—whether financial or ego-driven.

Step 4(c) Finding. Jane is in a period of her life in which many pediatricians would start to provide opportunities to meet with her privately for some portion of the clinical encounter. The pediatrician would explain the importance of this to her mother. We do not know enough about Jane's intellectual disability to tell whether she would be able to engage in these one-on-one conversations, but the presumption would be that she is developing her own degree of autonomy and individuality. More needs to be explored with regard to any familial or cultural issues that would have bearing on the situation. On the face of it, no concerns are raised about abuse or neglect—her mother seems to be making the request for OCP out of concern for her daughter's safety. As to whether the Mary's decision is challengeable, it depends on what harm the clinician is hoping to prevent. Use of an OCP is not associated with serious morbidity. There could be the question of whether being dishonest with the patient is a serious harm, especially if it undermines her trust in her mother, the pediatrician, and the health care system. This dignitary harm would have to be weighed against the harm of an unwanted pregnancy—harm reduction in the view of a colleague. A question has been raised by another colleague of whether one is legally required to follow the wishes of the parent, so it would be important to clarify what the legal parameters are (ie, when can the physician say "No" to a parent's request?). The case description does not suggest any institutional polices that are threatened. We also do not have evidence of the physician's position being influenced by any conflicts of interest or conflict of obligation.

CASE EVALUATION STEP 5
Are There Other Sources of Information that Can Provide Guidance to Help Resolve the Issue?

Once gathering and organizing the facts of a case, the clinician needs a means of determining their relevance in deriving possible solutions to an ethical concern. Common morality, principlism, or virtue theory may provide direction, but sometimes other methods of ethics analysis will prove useful.[47] Casuisitry is a method of practical ethics employing case-based reasoning.[48,49] It takes the particularities of a case and compares and contrasts them to a paradigm case. In reasoning by analogy, the judgment made in the paradigm case provides direction on how to settle the case at hand based on how similar or dissimilar it is to the values established by the paradigm. Because the casuistic method involves practical wisdom to discern how to apply maxims from previous cases, it is possible to see it as a complementary process to using reflective equilibrium to apply the prima facie principles of principlism to a case.[50] A similar process occurs in case law. In the legal system, cases are decided based on interpretation of the Constitution, established legislative law or statutes, or precedent cases—applying the law to the facts of a case.[51] In clinical medicine, case-based reasoning is common ("My current patient with diabetes is similar to a past patient with diabetes for whom I prescribed metformin and that patient did well, so I will prescribe metformin to my current patient"). So in the process of analyzing the facts in the ethics case analysis, the pediatrician should look for paradigm cases in ethics and/or the law.

Professional guidelines can be another means for clinicians to resolve an ethical concern. Professional societies publish codes, policies, position statements, and guidelines to educate their members on clinical issues in their field and set standards based on expert opinion and/or consensus votes by members. For instance, the American Medical Association has had a Code of Ethics since 1847, and its Council on Ethical and Judicial Affairs is responsible for maintaining and updating the Code for a variety of topics.[52] Within the American Academy of Pediatrics (AAP), "The Section on Bioethics provides pediatricians and pediatric subspecialists with an understanding of the basic principles of bioethics and promoting compassion, sensitivity, commitment, and high moral standards in the delivery of health care."[53] If a pediatrician is faced with a challenging case, checking to see if the AAP has addressed the issue could provide insights into how to manage the case.

Besides professional guidelines, books or journals may have addressed the issues involved in a patient's case. Medical textbooks may have chapters devoted to the topic or there may be clinical bioethics books that directly address the issue. Clinical or bioethics journals may have case reports, empirical research, reviews, or opinion pieces on the issue that the clinician is struggling with. Hotly debated issues are likely to have point and counterpoint articles, which can assist the clinician in thinking through the issue and making up their own mind based on the arguments presented. Stories on social media or in lay publications may also be influential.

Looking at a case with a different approach to ethics can expand the range of options considered by the pediatrician. Approaches like the ethic of care and narrative ethics are intentional about exploring the perspective of the parent or guardian and the child. The ethic of care shifts the focus from detached, impartial principles to relationships and attachment, recognizing the interdependence of involved parties.[54] Care ethics can be consonant with virtue ethics in that it concerns the skills and character traits of the one who cares.[55] Caring requires both conscientiousness and empathy.[56] The ethic of care challenges the carer (in this case, the pediatrician) to take responsibility for cultivating caring relationships and fostering social bonds and cooperation.[57] Relational ethical theory provides a foundation of "being-for" the patient.[37] Rather than assuming an impartial, abstract stance about the patient's personhood, the ethic of care requires the clinician to recognize the distinctive, concrete identity of the patient. A care orientation involves tapping into how the other person feels about their circumstances and being attuned to the contours of a situation. Discernment of the situation generates a caring response that might be different than one derived by application of principlism.[58]

Another approach to bioethics that differs from principlism is narrative ethics. A narrative approach involves framing the "characters" of the story and developing the plot—"the coherent ordering of a series of events" that lead to the story's ending and its meaning for all of the parties involved.[59] How the plot unfolds is dependent on who the narrator is and who the listeners are.[60] Narrative ethics holds that the patient is the ultimate author of their story and that the clinician helps to coauthor the patient's story by bearing witness to the patient's illness experience.[61] It may also require telling and retelling the story from different vantage points—backwards, sideways, and forward—to gain a richer understanding of the situation. Retelling a case helps to shape the moral considerations that should be brought to bear, seeing morality as an interpersonal task of making sense of the characters' lives and what ought to be done.[62] A narrative approach values dialogue "to help people tell stories that imagine the best possible ways to act."[63] In the end, "narrative saves deontology [duty-based ethics] from repeating abstractions that fail to recognize lived complexities."[64]

Step 5 Finding

Although Jane's case involves reversible contraception, the background on sterilization of children with developmental disabilities can be illuminating for both casuistry and attention to case law. The famous case of Carrie Buck who was involuntarily sterilized because of "feeblemindedness" led to an eventual backlash against eugenics in subsequent decades.[65] Laws in many states prohibit involuntary sterilization of persons with intellectual disability. Diekema argues that reproductive decisions for individuals with intellectual disability hinges on whether they have decision-making capacity and when they lack capacity that sterilization only proceed when adequate safeguards are in place (such as trying reversible forms of contraception first) and treatments are done in their best interests. In Jane's case, we do not have enough information to know whether she has decision-making capacity for reproductive health decisions. Another paradigmatic case to consider is giving high-dose estrogen to attenuate the growth of children with profound developmental disability.[66] Although it is not directly analogous to Jane's situation, the arguments used to support the parent's desire to define what is in their child's best interests can be examined to see if they have relevance to Jane's case.

As for professional guidelines, The American College of Obstetricians and Gynecologists has consensus statements on counseling adolescents about contraception and on medical management of menstrual suppression, including for those with cognitive disabilities.[67–69] With regard to whether Jane should be told what the OCP is for, the AAP policy on Informed Consent advocates for the assent of the patient and "helping the patient achieve a developmentally appropriate awareness of the nature of his or her condition" and "telling the patient what he or she can expect with tests and treatments."[30] In the ethics literature, one can find articles discussing truth telling and therapeutic privilege.[70,71] Truth telling takes on added complexity when cultural differences exist.[72,73] Guidelines and the literature seem to support the idea of discussing with Jane what is being prescribed in a developmentally appropriate and understandable manner.

As for the ethic of care and narrative ethics, the particularities of Jane's story are worthy of more exploration. Most notably, who is her mother and what is her story? The reader of the case will surmise that Mary was 15 year old when she became pregnant—what were the circumstances and does this explain why she is protective of her daughter? How would the story be told from the mother's perspective or from Jane's perspective? How does the pediatrician show care and concern in the therapeutic relationship while navigating this dilemma? Is there an opportunity for more discussion, rather than accepting Jane's mother's decision not to disclose the rationale for the OCP to Jane?

CASE EVALUATION STEP 6
What Are the Possible Options and what Action Will Be Taken?

After establishing the facts and analyzing them in terms of ethics frameworks, guidelines, or helpful literature, the next step is to decide on a course of action. Just as in clinical medicine where there may be a primary recommended treatment based on the medical evidence as well as alternatives that are perhaps not optimal but fall within the standard of care (including the option of no treatment if that is the patient's prerogative), the ethics analysis may yield a variety of options in how to proceed. Some options will be morally impermissible. Other options will be permissible but have their advantages and disadvantages based on the circumstances or which ethical approach, principle, or virtue is being highlighted. The pediatrician should employ the virtue of practical wisdom to discern between the options. One option may rise above the others for its ethical justification in what should be done. The arguments supporting this position should be coherent.[74] If at all possible, the preferable choice is the one to pursue, and the clinician needs moral courage to advocate for it. However, impediments may limit the choices of what can be done. Ultimately, clinical ethics is practical—a decision needs to be made of what will be done.

Step 6 Finding:
More information is needed in Jane's case before determining the range of options with regard to prescribing the OCP and what to tell Jane. The pediatrician can challenge the mother's stance about lying to Jane and explain the value of honesty and informing the patient. But it is important to first explore the reasons behind her mother not wanting to disclose the purpose. Greater understanding of the context is required.

CASE EVALUATION STEP 7
Once an Action Is Taken, What Are the Consequences? Does the Outcome Require a Re-Evaluation of the Plan?

As with clinical medicine when a treatment is instituted, the results of a course of action need to be evaluated. Were the anticipated benefits realized? Were there complications or unforeseen consequences? When uncertainty is a feature of the clinical decision, then sometimes a trial of therapy is recommended to provide more certainty of what the outcomes could be. Similarly, in clinical ethics, an opportunity exists to re-examine the decision based on how a case unfolds. Is more information learned over time that influences the pros and cons of the options available? The virtue of intellectual honesty entails that the clinician has humility not to remain fixed in their position but instead will adjust to new information or new ways of looking at an issue.

Step 7 Finding: The main course of action for the pediatrician to take in Jane's case is to continue the dialogue with her mother and encourage the participation of Jane in her own health care. Compassion and respect should be at the foundation of communication with Jane's mother, and the pediatrician should be open to what that discussion reveals.

DISCLOSURE STATEMENT WITH ANY COMMERCIAL OR FINANCIAL CONFLICTS OF INTEREST AND ANY FUNDING SOURCES

The author receives royalties as co-editor of *Curriculum Development for Medical Education: A Six-Step Approach* through The Johns Hopkins University Press 2022. The author receives royalties as a lecturer on clinical ethics through Lecturio (lecturio.com).

CONCLUSION

When a clinical case raises concerns for a pediatrician, a stepwise evaluation can help to determine the right course of action. The analysis involves identification of the ethical issues, organization of the main facts of the case, and selection of a morally permissible action after the tradeoffs of different options are assessed. It is important for the pediatrician to determine how much the minor patient can participate in the decision-making process and how best to preserve the therapeutic relationship between the pediatrician, parent, and child.

REFERENCES

1. Taylor HA, McDonald EL, Moon M, et al. Teaching ethics to paediatrics residents: the centrality of the therapeutic alliance. Med Educ 2009;43(10):952–9.
2. Moon M, Taylor HA, McDonald EL, et al. Everyday ethics issues in the outpatient clinical practice of pediatric residents. Arch Pediatr Adolesc Med 2009;163(9): 838–43.
3. Rushton CH, Kaszniak AW, Halifax JS. Addressing moral distress: application of a framework to palliative care practice. J Palliat Med 2013;16(9):1080–8.
4. Friedrich AB. The suffering child: claims of suffering in seminal cases and what to do about them. Pediatrics 2020;146(Suppl 1):S66–9.
5. Pellegrino ED. The internal morality of clinical medicine: a paradigm for the ethics of the helping and healing professions. J Med Philos 2001;26(6):559–79.
6. Bebeau MJ, Rest JR, Narvaez D. Beyond the promise: a perspective on research in moral education. Educ Res 1999;28(4):18–26.
7. You D, Bebeau MJ. The independence of James Rest's components of morality: evidence from a professional ethics curriculum study. Ethics Educ 2013;8(3): 202–16.
8. Cruess RL, Cruess SR, Boudreau JD, et al. A schematic representation of the professional identity formation and socialization of medical students and residents: a guide for medical educators. Acad Med 2015;90(6):718–25.
9. Clouser KD. Common morality as an alternative to principlism. Kennedy Inst Ethics J 1995;5(3):219–36.

10. Gert B. Introduction. In: Common morality: deciding what to do. New York: Oxford University Press; 2004. p. 7–12.

11. Foundation ABIM, Foundation ACP-ASIM. European Federation of Internal Medicine, European Federation of Internal Medicine. Medical professionalism in the new millennium: a physician charter. Ann Intern Med 2002;136(3):243–6.

12. Pellegrino ED. Professionalism, profession and the virtues of the good physician. Mt Sinai J Med 2002;69(6):378–84.

13. Pellegrino ED, Thomasma DC. *The virtues in medical practice*. Oxford: Oxford University Press; 1993.

14. Beauchamp TL, Childress JF. *Principles of biomedical ethics*. 8th Edition. Oxford: Oxford University Press; 2019.

15. Bolton J. What do we do when we "do" clinical ethics? A primer. J Clin Ethics, Spring 2023;34(1):110–5.

16. Centers for Disease Control and Prevention. Gateway to Health Communication: Preferred Terms for Select Population Groups & Communities. Available at: https://www.cdc.gov/healthcommunication/Preferred_Terms.html. Accessed October 15, 2023.

17. Beauchamp TL, Childress JF. Principles of Biomedical Ethics. 8th Edition. Oxford: Oxford University Press; 2019. p. 73–4.

18. FitzGerald C, Hurst S. Implicit bias in healthcare professionals: a systematic review. BMC Med Ethics 2017 Mar 1;18(1):19.

19. Jonsen AR, Siegler M, Winslade WJ. *Clinical ethics: a practical approach to ethical decisions in clinical medicine*. 9th Edition. New York: McGraw-Hill; 2022.

20. Steiner MJ, Trussell J, Johnson S. Communicating contraceptive effectiveness: an updated counseling chart. Am J Obstet Gynecol 2007;197(1):118.

21. Kuther TL. Medical decision-making and minors: issues of consent and assent. Adolescence 2003 Summer;38(150):343–58.

22. Coleman DL, Rosoff PM. The legal authority of mature minors to consent to general medical treatment. Pediatrics 2013;131(4):786–93.

23. Diekema DS. Adolescent brain development and medical decision-making. Pediatrics 2020;146(Suppl 1):S18–24.

24. Logan DE, Marlatt GA. Harm reduction therapy: a practice-friendly review of research. J Clin Psychol 2010;66(2):201–14.

25. Cardwell v Bechtol, 724 SW 2d 739, 745 (Tenn 1987).

26. McCabe MA. Involving children and adolescents in medical decision making: developmental and clinical considerations. J Pediatr Psychol 1996;21(4):505–16.

27. Mathews B. Adolescent capacity to consent to participate in research: a review and analysis informed by law, human rights, ethics, and developmental science. Laws 2023;12(1):2.

28. Sawyer K, Rosenberg AR. How should adolescent health decision-making authority be shared? AMA J Ethics 2020;22(5):E372–9.

29. Appelbaum PS. Clinical practice. assessment of patients' competence to consent to treatment. N Engl J Med 2007;357(18):1834–40.

30. Katz AL, Webb SA, AAP COMMITTEE ON BIOETHICS. Informed consent in decision-making in pediatric practice. Pediatrics 2016;138(2):e20161485.

31. Unguru Y. Making sense of adolescent decision-making: challenge and reality. Adolesc Med State Art Rev 2011;22(2):195–206, vii-viii.

32. Caplan AL. Challenging teenagers' right to refuse treatment. Virtual Mentor 2007; 9(1):56–61.

33. Bondi SA, Scibilia J. COMMITTEE ON MEDICAL LIABILITY AND RISK MANAGE-MENT. Dealing with the caretaker whose judgment is impaired by alcohol or drugs: legal and ethical considerations. Pediatrics 2019;144(6):e20193153.
34. Fanaroff JM, Committee on medical liability and risk management. Consent by Proxy for Nonurgent Pediatric Care. Pediatrics 2017;139(2):e20163911.
35. Lerand SJ. Teach the teacher: adolescent confidentiality and minor's consent. J Pediatr Adolesc Gynecol 2007;20(6):377–80.
36. Goldenring J, Rosen D. Getting into adolescent heads: an essential update. Contemp Pediatr 2004;21(1):64–90.
37. Furler JS, Palmer VJ. The ethics of everyday practice in primary medical care: responding to social health inequities. Philos Ethics Humanit Med 2010;5:6.
38. Committee on hospital care and institute for patient- and family-centered care. Patient- and family-centered care and the pediatrician's role. Pediatrics 2012; 129(2):394–404.
39. Committee on bioethics. Conflicts between religious or spiritual beliefs and pediatric care: informed refusal, exemptions, and public funding. Pediatrics 2013; 132(5):962–5.
40. Flaherty EG, Stirling J Jr, American Academy of Pediatrics. Committee on child abuse and neglect. clinical report—the pediatrician's role in child maltreatment prevention. Pediatrics 2010;126(4):833–41.
41. Diekema DS. Parental refusals of medical treatment: the harm principle as threshold for state intervention. Theor Med Bioeth 2004;25(4):243–64.
42. Diekema DS. Revisiting the best interest standard: uses and misuses. J Clin Ethics 2011 Summer;22(2):128–33.
43. Taylor M. Conceptual challenges to the harm threshold. Bioethics 2020;34(5): 502–8.
44. Birchley G. Harm is all you need? Best interests and disputes about parental decision-making. J Med Ethics 2016;42(2):111–5.
45. Jonsen AR, Siegler M, Winslade WJ. Preferences of Patients. In: Clinical ethics: a practical approach to ethical decisions in clinical medicine. 9th Edition. New York: McGraw-Hill; 2022. p. 53–114.
46. Bailey ZD, Krieger N, Agénor M, et al. Structural racism and health inequities in the USA: evidence and interventions. Lancet 2017;389(10077):1453–63.
47. Sulmasy DP, Sugarman J. The many methods of medical ethics (Or, thirteen ways of looking at a blackbird). In: Sugarman J, Sulmasy DP, editors. Methods in medical ethics. Washington, D.C.: Georgetown University Press; 2001. p. 3–18.
48. Jonsen AR. Casuistry as methodology in clinical ethics. Theor Med 1991;12(4): 295–307.
49. Jonsen AR. Casuistry. In: Sugarman J, Sulmasy DP, editors. Methods in medical ethics. Washington, D.C.: Georgetown University Press; 2001. p. 104–25.
50. Kuczewski M. Casuistry and principlism: the convergence of method in biomedical ethics. Theor Med Bioeth 1998;19(6):509–24.
51. Hodge JG, Gostin LO. Legal methods. In: Sugarman J, Sulmasy DP, editors. Methods in medical ethics. Washington, D.C.: Georgetown University Press; 2001. p. 88–103.
52. American Medical Association. Code of Ethics. Available at: https://code-medical-ethics.ama-assn.org/. Accessed April 3, 2023.
53. American Academy of Pediatrics. Section on Bioethics. 2023. Available at: https://www.aap.org/en/community/aap-sections/bioethics/. Accessed April 3, 2023.

54. Jecker NS, Reich WT. Care: III. Contemporary ethics of care. In: Post SG, editor. Encyclopedia of bioethics. 3rd edition. New York: Macmillan Reference USA; 2004. p. 367–73.
55. Carse AL. The 'voice of care': implications for bioethical education. J Med Philos 1991;16(1):5–28.
56. Tong R. The ethics of care: a feminist virtue ethics of care for healthcare practitioners. J Med Philos 1998;23(2):131–52.
57. Held V. The Ethics of Care as Moral Theory. In: The ethics of care: personal, political, and global. Oxford: Oxford University Press; 2005. p. 9–28.
58. Carse AL. Impartial principle and moral context: securing a place for the particular in ethical theory. J Med Philos 1998;23(2):153–69.
59. Charon R, Montello M. Framing the case: narrative approaches for healthcare ethics committees. HEC Forum 1999;11(1):6–15.
60. Chambers TS, Montgomery K. Plot: framing contingency and choice in bioethics. HEC Forum 1999;11(1):38–45.
61. Jones AH. Narrative based medicine: narrative in medical ethics. BMJ 1999; 318(7178):253–6.
62. Nelson HL. Context: backward, sideways, and forward. HEC Forum 1999;11(1): 16–26.
63. Frank AW. Narrative ethics as dialogical story-telling. Hastings Cent Rep 2014; 44(1 Suppl):S16–20.
64. Frank AW. Truth telling, companionship, and witness: an agenda for narrative ethics. Hastings Cent Rep 2016;46(3):17–21.
65. Diekema DS. Involuntary sterilization of persons with mental retardation: an ethical analysis. Ment Retard Dev Disabil Res Rev 2003;9:21–6.
66. Gunther DF, Diekema DS. Attenuating growth in children with profound developmental disability: a new approach to an old dilemma. Arch Pediatr Adolesc Med 2006;160(10):1013–7.
67. Counseling adolescents about contraception. Committee Opinion No. 710. American College of Obstetricians and Gynecologists. Obstet Gynecol 2017;130:e74–80.
68. American College of Obstetricians and Gynecologists' Committee on Clinical Consensus–Gynecology. General approaches to medical management of menstrual suppression: ACOG clinical consensus No. 3. Obstet Gynecol 2022; 140(3):528–41.
69. American College of Obstetricians and Gynecologists' Committee on Health Care for Underserved Women, Contraceptive Equity Expert Work Group, and Committee on Ethics. American college of obstetricians and gynecologists' committee on health care for underserved women, contraceptive equity expert work group, and committee on ethics. patient-centered contraceptive counseling: ACOG committee statement number 1. Obstet Gynecol 2022;139(2):350–3.
70. Cole CM, Kodish E. Minors' right to know and therapeutic privilege. Virtual Mentor 2013;15(8):638–44.
71. Richard C, Lajeunesse Y, Lussier MT. Therapeutic privilege: between the ethics of lying and the practice of truth. J Med Ethics 2010;36(6):353–7.
72. Unguru Y. Culturally aware communication promotes ethically sensitive care. Am J Bioeth 2022;22(6):31–3.
73. Rosenberg AR, Starks H, Unguru Y, et al. Truth telling in the setting of cultural differences and incurable pediatric illness: a review. JAMA Pediatr 2017;171(11): 1113–9.
74. Kaldjian LC, Weir RF, Duffy TP. A clinician's approach to clinical ethical reasoning. J Gen Intern Med 2005;20(3):306–11.

The Philosophical Underpinning of the Family for Pediatric Decision-Making

Lainie Friedman Ross, MD, PhD[a,b,c,d,*]

KEYWORDS

- Dyadic doctor–patient relationship • Triadic doctor–patient relationship
- Rights and responsibilities of parents • Pediatric decision-making

KEY POINTS

- Although traditional medical ethics focuses on the dyadic doctor–patient relationship, when the patient is a child, the relationship is triadic, meaning it involves the patient, the parent(s), and the clinician.
- A brief examination of the family, the rights and responsibilities of parents, the rights of children, and the moral basis of the parent–child relationship provide a philosophic underpinning for understanding the family in pediatric decision-making.
- Although biological parents have presumptive authority to make health-care decisions for their children, and are given wide discretion, parental autonomy is not absolute.
- Children have rights that require third parties (clinicians and/or the state) to intervene if their parents' decision falls below some threshold of abuse or neglect.

CASES

Case 1: Charlie Smith is a 4-day-old infant who presents to his pediatrician to establish care. Charlie was born at 39 3/7 weeks weighing 3.5 kg with Apgars of 8 and 9 at 1 and 5 minutes, respectively. While taking the family history, you learn that Charlie's father was diagnosed with retinoblastoma at 14 months and had his left eye enucleated. There is no other family history of childhood-onset conditions. You recommend genetic counseling and testing for RB1, the gene associated with retinoblastoma. Charlie's mother explains that they were offered and refused genetic testing in utero and do not want genetic testing now. You explain that the gene is autosomal dominant

[a] Department of Health Humanities and Bioethics, University of Rochester School of Medicine and Dentistry; [b] Department of Pediatrics, University of Rochester School of Medicine and Dentistry; [c] Paul M Schyve Center for Bioethics, University of Rochester; [d] Department of Philosophy, University of Rochester
* Corresponding author. University of Rochester Medical Center, 601 Elmwood Avenue, Box 676 (Room G-8011), Rochester, NY 14642.
E-mail address: Lainie_Ross@URMC.Rochester.edu

Pediatr Clin N Am 71 (2024) 27–37
https://doi.org/10.1016/j.pcl.2023.08.007
0031-3955/24/© 2023 Elsevier Inc. All rights reserved.

so there is a 50% chance that Charlie inherited the gene. If Charlie is known to have the gene, you would recommend frequent ophthalmologic evaluation in the first 5 years of life as Charlie has a very high likelihood of developing eye cancer, which if treated early, can be curative. If he does not have the gene, ophthalmologic screening would be unnecessary.

The Smiths are adamant that they do not want genetic testing. However, they are willing to have Charlie followed with frequent ophthalmologic evaluation. You explain that this potentially exposes Charlie to unnecessary evaluation, which by 9 months will require examination under anesthesia. They express understanding but insist on frequent ophthalmologic screening. Although not "best," is this good enough?

Case 2: Peter Dent is a 6-year-old boy who has been battling lymphoma for more than 2 years. His doctors discuss the current treatment options with his parents, and they decide together that the next treatment regimen will be a bone marrow transplant. The physicians find a "good" match (9 out of 10 human leukocyte antigen [HLA]-match) on the international bone marrow registry from a 30-year-old man, although they explain that a donation from a histoidentical family member would have the highest chance of success. All of Peter's family undergo HLA testing that same day. Peter's 3-year-old sister, Lisa, is found to be a perfect match. The parents authorize Lisa to serve as the stem cell donor and Peter's bone marrow transplant.

INTRODUCTION

The classic example of medical decision-making involves a clinician and an adult patient who has decision-making capacity. Although the relationship is classically thought of as dyadic—involving 2 parties—clinicians may have other team members engaged (eg, nurses and trainees) and patients can elect to include other individuals (family members or friends) in the process. Although adult patients usually have the right to accept or refuse all medical care, including life-saving medical care, there are exceptions to patient autonomy and the need for informed consent (eg, emergency care). However, in general, ultimate authority to accept or refuse a particular intervention, even life-saving intervention, belongs to the patient. If the patient lacks decisional authority, a surrogate is involved (either a proxy named by the patient when he/she had decisional capacity, or a surrogate determined by state health-care surrogacy ladders). The surrogate is supposed to act as the patient would have acted if he or she could speak for himself or herself (the principle of substituted judgment). If the patient's wishes are unknown, the surrogate is supposed to use a best interest standard.

When the patient is a child, the relationship is triadic, meaning it involves the patient, the parent(s), and the clinician. In general, parents have health-care decision-making authority for their minor children. There are exceptions (eg, when the child is emancipated due to parenthood or military service) as well as exceptional situations (eg, specialized consent statutes for contraceptive counseling). Traditional medical ethics asserts that parents should act in their child's best interest. The role of the minor, and when his or her assent is or should be sought depends on the age of the child, his or her maturity and decisional capacity, whether the clinical condition is life threatening or elective, and the treatment options that are available.

For most pediatric professionals in a liberal society (by which I mean a Western democracy), the above paragraphs cohere with what we were taught in medical ethics lectures. However, philosophers have been challenged by pediatric ethics and how to address the family and its minor children in models of pediatric decision-making. Historically, political philosophers were challenged by families because philosophy focuses on the public sphere, which Habermas defined as consisting of people who could meet and have critical debate about the needs of society with the state,[1] versus families which belong to the private sphere. Although principles of justice prevail in the public sphere, the family was perceived as a group (community) that is regulated by intimacy and caring—and as such, formal principles of justice were not necessary and could even be thought to hinder its functioning.[2] Feminist philosophers began to criticize the public/private distinction in the 1960s arguing that "The personal is political,"[3] and that the failure to apply principles of justice to the family leaves women and children vulnerable.[4]

Historically, there was little written in the philosophy literature about the parent–child relationship and what claims children might have against their parents (and/or the state). Philosophers were challenged by the involuntary nature of the family where children are dependent on third parties (parents or guardians) whom they did not choose. Philosophers also questioned whether biological parents caused "this needy being to exist" (causal agency) meant that parents should have primary childrearing responsibility.[5] If parents have duties to their children based on causal agency, these duties seem to be defeasible as parents could voluntarily relinquish their authority,[6] or involuntarily have their authority usurped.[7] If parents do not have duties based on causal agency,[5] philosophers wondered how to assign parental responsibilities because children are not capable of surviving, let alone be able to thrive without guardian support for more than a decade. Finally, philosophers were challenged by children because they were not full persons in the Kantian sense (of being fully rational beings)[8] and, therefore, did not (or should not have had) the same rights as adults. Joel Feinberg provided a typology of the different rights held by children and adults: (1) A-C rights, which are held by both adults and children (eg, the right not to be physically assaulted); (2) A rights, which are held only by autonomous adults (eg, the right to vote); and (3) C rights, which are held primarily by children.[8] C-rights include dependency rights— rights to certain goods that are owed because of the child's dependence on adults for the necessities of life.[8] This can also be framed as the difference between positive and negative rights. Although many A-rights are negative rights, which limit the actions of other persons or governments toward or against the right holder, such as the right to noninterference, C-rights focus on positive rights such as the provision of education, nutrition, and health care.

So, let us go behind the Oz curtain and examine the moral and philosophic issues that underpin the assumptions we routinely use in pediatric decision-making using the 2 cases described above: (1) whether to force Charlie's parents to authorize genetic testing and (2) whether to allow the Dents to authorize the stem cell donation of their young daughter to save her brother. We will examine 6 questions of political and moral philosophy: (1) What is meant by the concept "family"? (2) How are parents identified? (3) What is the moral basis of the parent–child relationship? (4) Why do parents have presumptive rights to raise their children according to their own values? (5) How do we define what is in a child's best interest? and (6) What are the limits to parental autonomy? After this philosophic examination, we will return to the 2 cases.

What Is Meant by the Concept "Family"?

There is no simple definition of the family, which takes many shapes and has variable size. The definition has also changed over time with changing laws about who can marry, the availability and social acceptability of divorce, and changing social mores about bearing and raising children outside of marriage. Some also distinguish between biological families (families of origin), which may not be biologic (whether due to adoption or the use of assisted reproductive technologies) versus families of choice. In the twenty-first century US society, there is a focus on the nuclear family but in other cultures, there may be greater focus on extended families.

Why does it matter who is or is not included in the family? It matters because most children are raised in families. It matters because children do not, contra the philosopher Hobbes, "spring out of the earth like mushrooms."[9] Rather, children are born quite needy and are dependent for years on one or more adults who "is capable of and responsible for providing for their "primary goods".[10(p5)] For the political philosopher John Rawls, "primary goods" are "things it is supposed a rational man wants, whatever else he wants."[11(pp 15-16)] Jeff Blustein enumerates what are the primary goods that parents must provide to their children: "Caretakers must protect children's health, develop the physical, emotional, and intellectual competences necessary to rational action, nourish their self-esteem and self-confidence, ready them to take advantage of and responsibly exercise their rights and liberties as citizens, and, as far as possible, provide them with conditions favorable to grasping educational, occupational, and other opportunities available to them in society."[12(pp. 124-5)]

How Are Parents Identified?

Traditional conceptions of parenthood focus on biology: parents are the biological creators of their progeny. However, the lines get blurry with some forms of assisted reproduction where biology can be split between genetic and gestational parents. Courts may then look to the "manifested intention" of being a parent.[13] Finally, parenthood could be fully separated from biology if biological parents relinquish their rights and other parents take on the rights and responsibilities (as in adoption). Moreover, although societies could be (and have been) organized where children are not raised (or at least are not exclusively raised) by their biological parents (eg, an Israeli kibbutz), most children in the United States are raised in households led by parent(s) or other adults who assume legal guardianship.

The assignment of parenthood is important because parents have presumptive right to raise the children that they bear, and they have the right to raise them according to their own values. However, with these rights come responsibilities: parents have primary responsibility to provide for their children's "primary goods," including the basic needs of food, shelter, and education. They do not do this alone because children are members of society, which means the state, through its *parens patria* function, also has responsibilities to help provide for these needs.

What Is the Moral Basis of the Parent–Child Relationship?

If parents have primary responsibility to provide for the primary goods of their children, then they must have both the authority and the resources to do so. At the extremes, there are 2 distinct interpretations of parental authority. At one extreme, children are perceived as the property of their parents who have virtually absolute power over them. At the other extreme, parents are perceived as fiduciaries of their children with duties to promote their best interest. Although children historically were considered property, today children are understood to be "rights holders," which limit parental authority. Some of these rights can be acted on in infancy (C-rights include the right to food and shelter) and other rights are rights-in-trust (A-rights, which will be granted to the child at some later age).[14]

Whether parents can be understood to be fiduciaries is complicated. A fiduciary is a person or organization who acts on behalf of another person and is bound both legally and ethically to act in the other's best interests.[15] Although it is often stated that parents are held to a best interest standard, in fact, they are not.[10,16] Consider the 2 cases above. Although it is in Charlie's best interest to have genetic testing done to determine what degree of follow-up is necessary, if Charlie's parents are willing to undergo quarterly eye examinations, most would say that their decision is "good enough." So clearly, they are not held to fiduciary standards. Moreover, although Peter's parents are clearly acting as his fiduciary when they authorize the testing of his siblings, it is not clear that it is in the best interest of his siblings to be tested. As such, the Dents may not be able to act in both of their children's best interest. Thus, parents do not, and often cannot, serve as fiduciaries to their child(ren).

If parents are not property owners of their children and are either not expected or are unable to be fiduciaries to their children, then what is the moral approach to the parent–child relationship? Jeffrey Blustein proposes the priority thesis, which holds that parental duties (responsibilities) take absolute priority over parental rights.[12] Parental duties derive from the parents' status as guardians of their children and include duties of need fulfillment (duties to protect a child's physical, emotional, and psychological development) and duties of respect (which includes "duties to respect a child's own desires and wants in matters not critical to protecting the child's basic interests").[12(p. 117)] Parental rights, however, accord parents certain freedoms and powers derived from their status as parents (which includes the freedom to raise their children according to their own conception of the good life) as well as the rights to fulfill their nonparental interests. According to the priority thesis, even if parents cannot always act in their child's best interest, they should still strive toward promoting their child's best interests, even at the expense of their own life projects.[12]

Ross rejects Blustein's priority thesis because it would demand that parents always place their child's physical and psychological development over their own needs and interests.[10] In *Children, Families and Health Care Decision-Making*, Ross describes the case of Amy Smith, a 9-year-old girl with cerebral palsy who would benefit from getting therapies at a rehabilitation center in a city 3 hours from where she lives with her parents.[10] Her parents may decide to go to a local rehabilitation center, even if they were informed that Amy's progress would be better if she attended the city-based center. Her parents may choose to remain in the countryside to fulfill their own projects (they may own a farm), for the projects of Amy's siblings (the schools may be better) or merely for lifestyle preferences. Ross argues that Amy's parents morally cannot neglect Amy's rehabilitative needs but they may balance better rehabilitative services with other needs and interests within the family.[10] Parents only have to make "good enough" decisions.

If parents are allowed to balance their own needs, interests, or preferences with the needs of their child, this implies that there are limits to parental responsibilities. Although parents have primary responsibility for providing for their child's primary goods, the quantity and type of a particular primary good will depend on the parents' beliefs, values, and conception of the good life. In liberal communities, the state tolerates a wide range of distributions among families provided that the parents provide their children with a threshold level of each primary good. "Parents require wide latitude to balance the health care needs of their child with the child's need for other primary goods, and with the needs and interests of other family members."[10(p. 8)] In this vein, then, it is morally permissible to permit Charlie's parents to refuse genetic testing provided they do consent for quarterly ophthalmologic evaluations. It is also permissible for the Dents to expose Lisa to the risks of a stem cell donation (but would not be permissible to expose Lisa to the risks of a living liver lobe donation) to benefit her sibling. Parents are required to promote their child's primary goods. They can make compromises against a primary good (health) as long as the donation does not reach a threshold of harm (often cited as a threshold of abuse or neglect).

Why Do Parents Have Presumptive Rights to Raise their Children According to their Own Values?

In their seminal work, *Deciding for Others: The Ethics of Surrogate Decision Making*, Allen Buchanan and Dan Brock describe why parents are allowed to make such compromises.[16] They argue that the underlying values that support a surrogate's decision-making for a formerly competent adult patient should focus first on the patient's interest in self-determination (determined using the principle of substituted judgment) and only second on well-being (best interest).[16] However, when the patient is a child, Buchanan and Brock change the order of underlying values—well-being is given primacy over self-determination and they add a third value, parental interests.[16] Buchanan and Brock provide 4 justifications for including parental interests as an underlying value: (1) "parents will usually do a better job of deciding than anyone else who could, as a general practice, be substituted for them"; (2) "parents must bear the consequences of treatment choices"; (3) "a right of parents, at least within limits, to raise their children according to the parents' own standards and values and to seek to transmit those standards and values to their children"; and (4) the value of the family as a social institution.[16(pp. 232–5)] Thus, parents are not fiduciaries whose only focus is on their child's best interests but they are individuals with their own goals and values, one of which is the sharing and inculcating of their beliefs to their progeny.

Three parenting styles were first described by Diana Baumrind at the University of California at Berkeley in the 1960s, and Eleanor Maccoby and John Martin added a fourth style in the 1980s. The 4 different parenting styles are as follows: permissive, authoritative, neglectful, and authoritarian.[17] Each style has different effect on a child's behavior. Although research suggests that authoritative parents are more likely to raise independent, self-reliant, and socially competent children,[18] it is also known that different children respond differently to different parenting styles and that one size does not fit all children or all situations. To the extent that we want to take parental interests seriously, we need to respect parents who do not want to raise independent children but would rather raise children who will adopt their cultural or religious values with minimal pushback (eg, the Amish). Because there is no consensus on what is the good life or how to measure it, we defer to parents about how they raise their children and this includes their right to be the presumptive decision makers for their child's health care (although the right is defeasible, for example, if their decision would reach a threshold of abuse or neglect). Enshrining parental decision-making in some zone of privacy also allows the parents to achieve their life goals as for many adults, bearing and/or rearing children is integral to their life plans.

How Do We Define What Is in a Child's Best Interest?

If parents are to be held to a best interest standard, then the child's best interest must be determinable. But is this the case? Let us take the case of the Dents. Although one assumes that it is in Charlie's best interest to undergo genetic testing as an infant to determine whether ophthalmologic follow-up is needed, this may not be the case. If the parents learn that Charlie is at risk, they may rear him differently than if they did not know his risk status. Data show that the "vulnerable child syndrome" can be harmful to his emotional and psychological development.[19,20] Similarly, one assumes that it is in Peter's best interest to get a bone marrow donation from his sister but the fact is that the stem cells may not graft. Depending on how the stem cells are collected and stored, and the quantity obtained, they may be less effective than one might have hoped. Similarly, if Peter does get undergo a successful stem cell transplant, it may be that he feels beholden to his sister for saving his life and this leads to feelings of low self-esteem and anger which has a deleterious effect on his relationships with his sibling and his parents.

So how do we determine what is in a child's best interest? More specifically, if we are using best interest as a guidance principle for health-care decision-making, do we consider what is in a child's best interest, all things considered or just focus on what is in a child's medical best interest?[16] Moreover, even if we agree on which factors to include in a best interest calculation, people can prioritize different interests differently and therefore reach different conclusions about what is best.[21] It is also not clear whether one must focus exclusively on the child's self-regarding interests versus whether the calculation can include other-regarding interests. A narrow focus on self-regarding interests ignores the fact that children are members of a family, and as John Hardwig argues, "There is no way to detach the lives of patients from the lives of those who are close to them. Indeed, the intertwining of lives is part of the very meaning of closeness."[22(p. 5)] Further, Ross argues that an exclusive focus on self-regarding best interests denies the need to consider parental values, needs, and interests; the right of parents to raise their child according to their own values, even if those values are not perceived as "best" by others; and the need to balance children's best interests when parents have more than one child.[10]

What Are the Limits of Parental Autonomy?

In a liberal society, parents expect to raise their children free from state intervention.[23] However, this does not mean that they can do anything they want; Buchanan and Brock offer several other scenarios where parental autonomy is constrained: "(1) disqualification of the surrogates based on abuse or neglect; (2) a requirement of special scrutiny for certain types of cases due to vulnerability" (such as individuals who are long-term residents of institutions, or decisions to procure organs or tissues from minors); and (3) a requirement that the decision "must be within the range of medically sound alternatives, as determined by appropriate medical community standards."[16(p. 143)]

In Ross' model of pediatric decision-making, constrained parental autonomy restricts parental autonomy based on the principle of respect for persons.[10] Respect for persons has both negative and positive components. The negative component holds universally and prohibits the abuse neglect and exploitation of all children. The positive component only holds in particular relationships (such as within the intimate family) and compels these particular individuals to provide particular children with the goods, skills, liberties, and opportunities necessary to become autonomous adults capable of devising and implementing their own life plans. A major difference between the model of constrained parental autonomy and a model based on the best interest standard is that the former model can accommodate intrafamilial trade-offs provided that the basic needs of each child member is secured.[10] So, the Dents can authorize Lisa's stem cell donation motivated by their desire to help Peter but cognizant that it may fail and cognizant of the risks (mostly transient harms) to which their decision exposes Lisa. Their decision is within their realm of discretion, regardless of the outcome.

RESOLUTION OF THE 2 CASES
Case 1

Because Charlie has a 50% chance of inheriting the RB1 gene, it is in Charlie's medical best interest to undergo genetic testing to determine if he has RB1. Charlie's parents refuse testing but believe they are acting in Charlie's best interest, all things considered. The physician should try to understand how the Smiths came to their decision. He should make sure they understand what is being proposed, correct misinformation, and address misconceptions. The physician should make sure that the Smiths understand he is focused on identifying whether Charlie has inherited a particular gene that requires early attention and that he is not recommending whole genome sequencing, which could uncover other genetic risk factors that may not be relevant to Charlie's short-term health or that only identify an increased statistical risk—the RB1 gene is virtually 100% penetrant in the first few years of life. The physician should try to understand the Smith's concerns—whether the parents fear unintended consequences of labeling Charlie as a carrier or the fear of its impact on their health insurance premiums. If the latter, he should education them about The Genetic Information Nondiscrimination Act of 2008 which prohibits discrimination on the basis of genetic information with respect to health insurance and employment.[24]

If Charlie's parents continue to refuse genetic testing, Charlie could undergo frequent eye evaluations. This is not medically best because it exposes some children to unnecessary evaluation, which may need to take place under general anesthesia and its attendant risks.[25] However, most clinicians would acknowledge that frequent eye evaluation is "good enough" or at least does not reach the threshold of abuse or neglect. However, if the Smiths refuse eye screening or fail to attend these appointments, then the physician may feel obligated to report this to child protective services on the grounds that Charlie has a 50% chance of having an eye cancer that can be successfully treated if diagnosed early but can be deadly if diagnosis and treatment are delayed.

Case 2

Consider the decision-making complexity confronting the parents of Peter and Lisa. Peter needs a bone marrow transplant, and getting stem cells from his sibling offers him the highest chance of survival (although without a guarantee). A stem cell donation from a stranger has the benefit that the adult can give his own informed consent to serve as a living donor, whereas Lisa is too young to understand and her parents must decide on her behalf. It may be in Lisa's best interest if Peter were to get a stem cell donation from the registry volunteer and thus avoid the risks of stem cell donation. Her risks may depend on the source of stem cells. Bone marrow donation is painful, requires anesthesia, and may lead to nerve damage or a need for a blood transfusion.[26,27] Peripheral stem cell collection involves large bore catheters and has a small risk of adverse events such as blood clots or infection. To increase the number of peripheral stem cells procured, donors are pretreated with granulocyte-colony stimulating factor, which can cause bone pain, headache, and flu-like symptoms.[28] Some children need blood transfusions after stem cell collection.[27]

Lisa's parents are also the decision-maker for her brother. It is in Peter's best interest to get a stem cell donation from his sister because the likelihood of success is greater when there is a sibling histoidentical match. One could say, then, that there is a conflict of interests—what is best for one may not be the best for the other.

Alternatively, one could argue that it is in both Peter's and Lisa's best interest for Lisa to be the stem cell donor because it gives Peter the best chance of success and Peter's well-being is integral to the family's well-being.[10,16] However, although Lisa's stem cell donation may be best for survival, the transplant may have unintended consequences. During adolescence and beyond, Peter may feel anger at his sister because she reminds him that he was ill and she gave a gift that he cannot repay. Conversely, if Peter were to do poorly, Lisa may blame herself when she is older for not providing the cure.

Clearly, the outcomes are unknowable and the Dents must make a decision under uncertainty. If the Dents believe that Peter's survival is best for Peter and for the family as a whole, then his parents should authorize the donation from Lisa to maximize Peter's chance of success. The risks to Lisa are small. However, the parents should be aware of the data that show that being a donor can cause serious psychological harm.[29–32]

There are ways to mitigate these risks. The American Academy of Pediatrics (AAP) Committee on Bioethics policy statement entitled "Children as Hematopoietic Stem Cell Donors" proposed including a donor advocate for all pediatric stem cell transplants to ensure that the donor's well-being is considered independently and that the concerns and needs of the potential child donor are addressed.[33] One point emphasized in the AAP statement is that the decision to do HLA testing should not be seen as a simple blood test that can be done automatically because the implications are anything but simple.[33] That seems to have been overlooked in this case but the donor advocate should get involved now and help prepare Lisa for the upcoming stem cell collection or bone marrow aspiration. Nondonor siblings may also require support as the data show that they often feel neglected as the focus is on the sick sibling and the potential savior donor.[30,34] The nondonor siblings may feel neglected or jealous that they were not the chosen one, or they may feel guilty because they feel relieved not to have been chosen.[30,34]

SUMMARY

A philosophic examination of the family, the rights and responsibilities of parents, the rights of children, and the moral basis of the parent–child relationship provide a philosophic underpinning for understanding pediatric decision-making. Although biological parents have presumptive authority to make health-care decisions for their children and are given wide discretion, parental autonomy is not absolute. Children have rights that require third parties (clinicians and/or the state) to intervene if their parents' decision falls below some threshold of abuse or neglect. Further examination of family obligations in health-care decision-making is needed and should include a discussion of the duties, if any, of children to their parents, of siblings across the life span, and to family members beyond the nuclear family.

CLINICS CARE POINTS

- The state should only intervene in parental decision-making when the decision is abusive or neglectful, not when the decision is good but there are better alternatives.
- Although it is often said that parents must act in their child's best interest, they are given much wider discretion and their decisions should not be overriden unless they are abusive or neglectful.

DISCLOSURE

The author has nothing to disclose.

REFERENCES

1. Habermas J. The Structural Transformation of the public sphere: an Inquiry into a category of Bourgeois society. Translated by Thomas Burger with Frederick Lawrence. Cambridge, MA: MIT Press; 1991.

2. Olsaretti, Serena. Family and Justice in Political Philosophy. Oxford Research Encyclopedias, Politics. March 25, 2021. Available at: https://oxfordre.com/politics/display/10.1093/acrefore/9780190228637.001.0001/acrefore-9780190228637-e-1766. Last accessed September 22, 2023.

3. Hanisch, C. "The Personal Is Political", The women's liberation movement classic with a new explanation. Available at: http://www.carolhanisch.org/CHwritings/PIP.html. Last accessed September 22, 2023.

4. Okin SM. Justice, Gender, and the family. New York: Basic Books; 1989.

5. Blustein J. On the Duties of Parents and Children. South J Philos 1977;15(4):427–41.

6. Nelson JL. Parental Obligations and the Ethics of Surrogacy: A Causal Perspective. Publ Aff Q 1991;5(1):49–61.

7. Child Welfare Information Gateway. (2021). Grounds for involuntary termination of parental rights. U.S. Department of Health and Human Services, Administration for Children and Families, Children's Bureau. Available at: https://www.childwelfare.gov/topics/systemwide/laws-policies/statutes/groundtermin/. Last accessed September 22, 2023.

8. Kant I. The metaphysics of morals. Translated by. M. Gregor. New York: Cambridge University Press; 1991.

9. Hobbes T. Man and citizen (De Homine and De cive). Indianapolis (IN): Hackett Publishing Company, Inc.; 1991.

10. Ross LF. Children, families, and health care decision-making. Oxford (UK): Oxford University Press; 1998.

11. Rawls J. A theory of justice. Cambridge (MA): Belknap Press of Harvard University Pres; 1971.

12. Blustein Je. Parents and children: the ethics of the family. New York: Oxford University Press; 1982.

13. Douglas G. The Intention to be a Parent and the Making of Mothers. Mod Law Rev 1994;57:636–41.

14. Feinberg J. The Child's Right to an Open Future. In: Aiken W, LaFollette H, editors. Whose child? Totowa (NJ): Rowman & Littlefield; 1980. p. 124–53.

15. Kagan J. Fiduciary Definition: Examples and Why it is Important. Investopedia.com. Updated September 15, 2022. Available at: https://www.investopedia.com/terms/f/fiduciary.asp#:~:text=A%20fiduciary%20is%20a%20person,in%20the%20other's%20best%20interests. Last accessed September 22, 2023.

16. Buchanan A, Brock D. Deciding for Others: the ethics of surrogate decision making. New York: Cambridge University Press; 1989.

17. Jessup University. The Psychology behind different types of parenting styles. Available at: https://jessup.edu/blog/academic-success/the-psychology-behind-different-types-of-parenting-styles/#:~:text=In%20the%201960s%2C%20psychologist%20Diana,Eleanor%20Maccoby%20and%20John%20Martin. Last accessed September 22, 2023.

18. Baumrind D. Authoritative Parenting Revisited: History and Current Status. In: Authoritative parenting: Synthesizing nurturance and discipline for optimal child development. 1st edition. Washington, DC: American Psychological Association; 2012. p. 11–34.

19. Green M, Solnit AJ. Reactions to the threatened loss of a child: A vulnerable child syndrome. Pediatric management of the dying child, part III. Pediatrics 1964;34:58–66.

20. Verbeek INE, van Onzenoort-Bokken L, Zegers SHJ. Vulnerable child syndrome in everyday paediatric practice: A condition deserving attention and new perspectives. Acta Paediatr 2021;10(2):397–9.
21. Rhodes R, Holzman IR. Is the best interest standard good for pediatrics? Pediatrics 2014;134(Suppl 2):S121–9.
22. Hardwig J. What about the Family? Hastings Cent Rep 1990;20(2):5–10.
23. Inness JC. Privacy, intimacy, and Isolation. New York: Oxford University Press; 1992.
24. Genetic Information Nondiscrimination Act of 2008. Public Law 110-233. Approved May 21, 2008.
25. Paterson N, Waterhouse P. Risk in pediatric anesthesia. Paediatr Anaesth 2011; 21(8):848–57.
26. Bosi A, Bartolozzi B. Safety of bone marrow stem cell donation: a review. Transplant Proc 2010;42(6):2192–4.
27. Styzcynski J, Balduzzi A, Gil L, et al. on behalf of the European Group for Blood and Marrow Transplantation Pediatric Diseases Working Party. Risk of complications during hematopoietic stem cell collection in pediatric sibling donors: a prospective European Group for Blood and Marrow Transplantation Pediatric Diseases Working Party study. Blood 2012;119(12):2935–42.
28. Pulsipher MA, Nagler A, Iannone R, et al. Weighing the Risks of G-CSF Administration, Leukopheresis, and Standard Marrow Harvest: Ethical and Safety Considerations for Normal Pediatric Hematopoietic Cell Donors. Pediatr Blood Cancer 2005;46(4):422–33.
29. Packman W, Weber S, Wallace J, et al. Psychological effects of hematopoietic SCT on pediatric patients, siblings and parents: a review. Bone Marrow Transplant 2010;45(7):1134–46.
30. Packman WL, Crittenden MR, Schaeffer E, et al. Psychosocial consequences of bone marrow transplantation in donor and nondonor siblings. Journal of Developmental & Behavioral Pediatrics 1997;18(4):244–53.
31. Pentz RD, Alderfer MA, Pelletier W, et al. Unmet needs of siblings of pediatric stem cell transplant recipients. Pediatrics 2014;133(5):e1156–62.
32. Wiener LS, Steffen-Smith E, Fry T, et al. Hematopoietic Stem Cell Donation in Children: a review of the sibling donor experience. J Psychosoc Oncol 2007;25(1): 45–66.
33. American Academy of Pediatrics Committee on Bioethics. Policy Statement: Children as Hematopoietic Stem Cell Donors. Pediatrics 2010;125(2):392–404.
34. Çoban ÖG, Adanır AS, Özatalay E. Post-traumatic stress disorder and health-related quality of life in the siblings of the pediatric bone marrow transplantation survivors and post-traumatic stress disorder in their mothers. Pediatr Transplant 2017;21(6):e13003.

Shared Decision-Making in Pediatrics

Kimberly E. Sawyer, MD, MA, HEC-C[a],*, Douglas J. Opel, MD, MPH[b,c]

KEYWORDS

- Pediatric • Shared decision-making • Framework • Bioethics • Standard of care
- Standard practice • Benefit • Burden

KEY POINTS

- Pediatric SDM should occur between clinicians and parents when a medical decision for a child has more than 1 medically reasonable management option.
- SDM exists on a continuum and includes both clinician-guided and parent-guided types. The type of SDM used depends on the medical benefit-burden ratio of the medically reasonable options, how preference-sensitive the options are to the parents, and other contextual features.
- Since there are some common patient-centered and family-centered communication strategies shared among several decision-making models in pediatrics, it can be confusing which decision-making model is being used. It is therefore important to be clear which model is indicated and why.

INTRODUCTION

Shared decision-making (SDM) has become an integral part of patient-centered and family-centered care. Many view it as the middle ground between clinician paternalism and patient consumerism. One definition of SDM, in fact, is "a collaborative process that allows patients, or their surrogates, and clinicians to make health care decisions together, taking into account the best scientific evidence available as well as the patient's values, goals, and preferences.[1]"

Pediatric SDM is distinct in part because the child patient is not yet a competent adult with whom a pediatric clinician can share a decision. Therefore, the intended beneficiary of SDM—the child patient—does not have the capacity to fully share in the decisions that affect his/her interests. Rather, to conduct pediatric SDM, clinicians

[a] Department of Pediatrics, Baylor College of Medicine, Texas Children's Hospital Palliative Care Team, 6621 Fannin Street, Suite W.1990, Houston, TX 77030, USA; [b] Department of Pediatrics, School of Medicine, University of Washington, Seattle, WA, USA; [c] Treuman Katz Center for Pediatric Bioethics, Seattle Children's Research Institute, 1900 9th Avenue, JMB 6, Seattle, WA 98101, USA
* Corresponding author. Texas Children's Hospital Palliative Care Team, 6621 Fannin Street, Suite W.1990, Houston, TX 77030, USA
E-mail address: kesawyer@texaschildrens.org

Pediatr Clin N Am 71 (2024) 39–48
https://doi.org/10.1016/j.pcl.2023.08.001
0031-3955/24/© 2023 Elsevier Inc. All rights reserved.
pediatric.theclinics.com

must engage with the child's surrogate decision maker (a parent or legal guardian) and elicit what the surrogate deems is in the child's, and potentially family's, best interest. SDM gets even more complex as the pediatric patient ages and it becomes less justifiable to exclude the child from decision-making out of respect for the child's emerging autonomy.

Pediatric SDM is also distinct because pediatric clinicians themselves, like parents, have an obligation to promote the child's best interest. This can constrain how shared a decision is with parents. For instance, eliciting parents' preferences, a hallmark of SDM, usually occurs in tandem with the clinician scrutinizing whether parents' preferences serve the child's best interest. Though others in this volume address ways to address the conflict that arises when surrogates and clinicians differ in their conceptions of what constitutes the child's best interest,[2–4] it nonetheless is clear that implementation of SDM in pediatrics presents unique challenges because it must accommodate multiple goals. Unlike in SDM with adults that is singularly focused on promoting patient autonomy, SDM in pediatrics must take into account protecting the child, honoring the emerging autonomy of adolescents, and respecting parental values and decision-making authority.

The authors have previously described a 4-step process for pediatric SDM.[5,6] This process is intended for clinicians facing any discrete decision in the medical care of a young child (as noted earlier, pediatric SDM with adolescents will likely require a different process). Briefly, the steps of the process encourage clinicians to determine (1) if there is more than 1 medically reasonable option (with steps 2–4 only applicable for decisions with >1 option, as these are the domains of SDM), (2) if 1 option has a favorable medical benefit-burden ratio, (3) how preference-sensitive the options are to the family, and (4) contextual features to help refine exactly how shared the decision should be (**Fig. 1**).

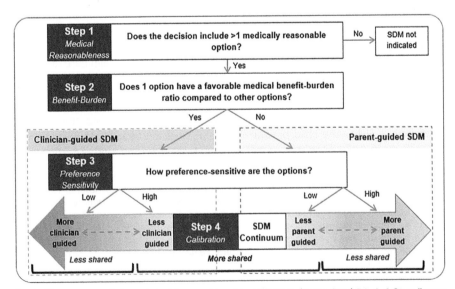

Fig. 1. The process of shared decision-making in pediatrics. (*From* Opel DJ. A 4-Step Framework for Shared Decision-making in Pediatrics. Pediatrics 2018;142(Suppl 3):S149-S56 https://doi.org/10.1542/peds.2018-0516E.)

The 4-step process for SDM in pediatrics was based on conceptual work on SDM in the adult setting, with adjustments to account for the aforementioned unique aspects of pediatric decision-making.[7–21] It has been found to be salient to parents and clinicians across a range of clinical scenarios. After videotaped encounters, investigators conducted individual postencounter interviews with clinician and parent participants that utilized video-stimulated recall to facilitate reflection of the decision-making that occurred during the encounter. Qualitative analysis of the interview transcripts found that clinicians' and parents' experiences of decision-making confirmed each SDM step.[22]

In this article, the objective is to briefly review the 4-step process, address difficulties with determining whether SDM should occur (Step 1), and comment on how the SDM process relates to, and may be conflated with, other decision-making models that may leverage some similar patient-centered and family-centered communication strategies.

DISCUSSION
Shared Decision-Making Process

Step 1: medical reasonableness
The first step in the process of implementing SDM is to consider whether there is more than 1 medically reasonable option to manage the clinical situation. If there is only 1 medically reasonable option, SDM is not indicated because there is not a decision to share. These scenarios necessitate a different decision-making approach for engaging with the parent about the 1 medically reasonable option, such as clinician-controlled decision-making.

Critical to the implementation of this step is defining medically reasonable. The authors propose that medically reasonable options are those that meet the standard of care (SOC). The SOC itself is defined as "minimally competent care" that other clinicians would provide under the same circumstances.[23–25] Ideally, interventions become the SOC because their safety and efficacy profiles are supported by quality scientific evidence, or in the absence of such evidence, by expert consensus. Professional guidelines are 1 source of SOC,[26,27] although such guidelines are not available for every potential clinical scenario. When there is no consensus about what the SOC is for a given clinical scenario, this, in general, is an indication that more than 1 medically reasonable option likely exists and SDM is appropriate.

It is also helpful in implementing this step to differentiate the SOC from standard practice. In general, standard practice represents "the widely agreed upon, state-of-the-art, high-quality level of practice" at an institution.[28] In this way, standard practice may be synonymous with the SOC. However, standard practice may also exceed the SOC, incorporating emerging data, organization-level expertise, or advanced technologies.[28] Standard practice may even vary by institution depending on availability of state-of-the-art information, experience, or equipment.

The importance of distinguishing standard practice from the SOC is evident when standard practice at an organization for a particular clinical situation exceeds that of the SOC. In these situations, it may appear, for instance, that there is only 1 medically reasonable option—the option that is consistent with standard practice—when in fact the standard practice exceeds the SOC and other options that meet the SOC exist. If this goes unrecognized, clinicians could mistakenly exclude medically reasonable options that conform to the SOC and not use SDM when they should.

Clinicians must also be mindful of how their own biases and values can influence their determination of what is medically reasonable. Some clinicians, for instance, may view a clinical scenario with multiple medically reasonable options as really having only 1 option because their own preference for a particular option limits their view of the full range of options. For example, evidence suggests that clinicians rank quality of life of children with chronic neurologic conditions lower than do children and parents.[29–31] This, in turn, may influence how clinicians approach decisions around code status or long-term life-sustaining technologies such as a tracheostomy and mechanical ventilation. Inappropriately limiting the option set could also occur due to our susceptibility as humans to use cognitive shortcuts, or heuristics, such as availability bias: we may exclude a medically reasonable option because our most recent or memorable patient had significant side effects or poor response to a therapy.[32]

Step 2: benefit-burden

If a clinical scenario has more than 1 medically reasonable option, it is appropriate to engage in SDM with the parent or legal guardian of the child patient. In step 2 of the SDM process, the medical benefit-burden ratio for each option is considered. This step is justified by clinician obligations to act in the best interest of the child. While parents are expected to make decisions that maximize benefits and minimize harm to the child, clinicians too have an obligation to ensure this by helping guide the maximizing of benefits and minimizing of harm. When there appears to be a favorable option, a clinician-guided SDM is appropriate. When there is no favorable option, it is appropriate to allow the parent to assume a more directive role (parent-guided SDM).

In determining whether there is a favorable option, it is most ideal if clinicians consider the probability and magnitude of the benefits and burdens of the medically reasonable options, as well as how certainly we may know those probabilities and magnitudes. Similar to step 1, clinicians should aim to be objective in their assessments of the benefits and burdens. They should also acknowledge that their own values and preferences related to risk tolerance may make this determination subjective and susceptible to bias. While it can still be appropriate to base a favorability assessment on personal experience or expert opinion when there is a lack of quality evidence to support a benefit-burden ratio determination, this should be acknowledged in discussions with the parent, and clinicians should resist making strong recommendations in these situations.

Step 3: preference sensitivity

Step 3 helps ensure parent preferences regarding the available options that are known and explored in order to align the chosen option with their values. Parents have the right and responsibility to make choices related to their children's medical care: they know their children the best, are permitted to instill their values in their children, and are best positioned to balance competing family interests. Therefore, even when 1 option is preferred by a clinician because of a more medically favorable benefit-burden ratio, "the best choice depends on how [the parent] values the risks and benefits of the treatments available.[33]"

Parents may not always have strong preferences or a preference at all. This step accommodates these different scenarios. For instance, in scenarios where parents do not have strong preferences regarding the available options in the setting where a clinician does have a favored option based on an assessment of the medical benefit and burdens of the available options, a more clinician-guided SDM approach is justifiable. Alternatively, if parents do have strong preferences for a particular option, and this differs from the clinician-favored option, a less clinician-guided SDM approach is warranted in favor of reaching a mutual decision aligned with the parent's values and preferences.

An important aspect of this step is going beyond simply asking the parent what they would like to do. Instead, implementing this step is meant to include engaging parents in articulating, exploring, and even constructing their preferences. This is justifiable since what we value and prefer as humans is an ongoing process subject to our capacity for change and self-reflection. Parents with clear goals, values, and preferences, for instance, may find themselves in a novel situation—such as a hospitalized child with a newly diagnosed chronic condition—and not only be unsure of how to apply their known values to the medical decisions at hand, but also may realize previous values and preferences require revision going forward. Furthermore, this process of change and self-reflection is often achieved through dialogue and discussion with others, including with clinicians.[34] This more expansive role for clinicians is, in fact, consistent with the first conceptions of SDM by the President's Commission for the Study of Ethical Problems in Medicine and Biomedical and Behavioral Research in which "an appropriate balance" was sought between patient autonomy and clinicians' obligation to promote patients' health and well-being.[35] Helping parents assess the worthiness of their health-related values is not manipulation or coercion.

The intent of this step is not to simply seek agreement with the clinician's favored option. Assuming parent preferences are being elicited if parents simply agree with the clinician's recommendation falls short of SDM. However, in recent observational work, investigators found several clinicians practicing SDM by eliciting parent preferences via making a recommendation and asking whether parents agree (eg, "Let's do this, sound ok?"), without pursuing further discussion if parents responded affirmatively.[22] It is apparent that how step 3 is operationalized is critical to the quality of SDM achieved.

Step 4: calibration

The final step is to determine a specific SDM approach on a continuum from clinician-guided to parent-guided. Depending on the medical benefit-burden ratio (step 2) and parent preferences (step 3), a decision may be appreciably guided by the clinician, the parent, or be more mutually shared. Additionally, other decisional factors may be used to calibrate the SDM approach, such as how quickly the decision must be made, whether the intervention is singular or repeated over time, and who will implement the intervention (clinician or parent). If these characteristics are present, they can justify changing the SDM approach from the one initially suggested by the answers to steps 2 and 3. For instance, management options that are longitudinal and parent-implemented, such as home-based treatment of a chronic disease, require more compliance and responsibility from parents, and therefore, despite answers to steps 2 and 3, the SDM approach in these circumstance may be calibrated to be more parent-guided (eg, if a decision was initially suggested to be clinician-guided, it would become more parent-guided). As parents gain more experience and expertise about their child's health and treatment, decisions that were more shared may also shift to becoming more parent-guided over time. Conversely, for medically reasonable options that are clinician-implemented, such as whether ketamine or propofol sedation is used for fracture reduction in the emergency department, it may be acceptable to move toward a more clinician-guided approach despite the SDM approach suggested from the answers to steps 2 and 3 given how important role of clinician experience with administering these medications is in this decision.

How the Shared Decision-Making Process Relates to Other Models of Decision-Making

SDM ought to be recognized as a specific approach to medical decision-making. Here, the authors clarify how SDM relates to and differs from other models of decision-making (**Fig. 2**). Attending to these differences is critical to the implementation of SDM.

Overlapping Communication Strategies

SDM can be confused with other models of pediatric decision-making because it shares some communication methods with other models. For instance, SDM and many other decision-making models include use of collaborative communication techniques with patients and families, such as active listening, reflection, and affirmation statements. Use of these techniques is so prevalent because they can deepen rapport, improve engagement, and help parents feel understood, common goals in nearly all decision-making. Therefore, presence or use of these techniques does not necessarily mean that the process being used is SDM. Clinician-controlled decision-making may incorporate these techniques too, for instance, but as a means to understand more about a parent's reluctance to accept the 1 medically reasonable option. Therefore, it is essential not to conflate the use of collaborative communication strategies as necessarily doing SDM.

When Parents Decline all Medically Reasonable Options

Parents may not accept the medically reasonable option or options, and it may seem appropriate to allow this refusal to influence whether SDM is used. Indeed, investigators found evidence that, at times, clinicians hinged their determinations of whether there is more than 1 option—and therefore whether to use SDM—on whether they would honor a parent's refusal of the 1 medically reasonable option.[22] This, however, is problematic because whether an option is medically reasonable and whether a parent's refusal of a medically reasonable option should be respected require different considerations. Whether an option is medically reasonable should be informed by clinical evidence and SOC. Conversely, whether a parent's refusal of that option would be honored is based on the risk of harm to the child, as described in the Harm Principle.[19]

Consider 2 scenarios. The first involves a parent refusing an urgent (but not emergent) blood transfusion for their child who has severe anemia. The second is a parent refusing a recommended vaccine for their otherwise healthy child. Both represent situations in which there is 1 medically reasonable option based on the SOC, and therefore SDM is not appropriate. However, in the first scenario, it would be appropriate to contact child protective services given the significant risk of serious harm to the child by the parent's refusal (compared to receipt of a blood transfusion). In the second scenario, referral to child protective services would be less justifiable, given the low risk of serious harm (though not zero) to the child by remaining unimmunized. Integrating determinations of what is medically reasonable with determinations of whether parent refusal would be honored could result in the use of SDM when it is not appropriate.

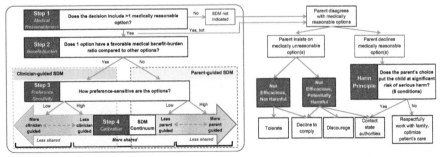

Fig. 2. How shared decision-making relates to other models of decision-making.

When Parents Request Medically Unreasonable Options

Occasionally, parents will request and insist on therapies that do not meet the SOC and therefore are not medically reasonable. These can range from complementary and integrative medicine modalities (including herbs, supplements, and energy-based therapies) to life-sustaining therapies (such as mechanical ventilation) in situations of physiologic futility. There are a broad range of potential appropriate responses to these requests.

If there is potential benefit to the therapy, then it is appropriate to consider the parent's suggestion under the SDM process as a medically reasonable option. If the suggested therapy is not efficacious (based on negative or lack of evidence) but is also not harmful, and the parent administers the therapy without action needed on the part of the clinician, then it is reasonable to tolerate the parent's request. If it is not efficacious but also not harmful and the clinician is being asked to administer an intervention, clinicians may decide that additional benefits accrued through relationship-building may warrant complying with the request. Alternatively, clinicians may consider the cost, resources, experience, or other considerations required to comply with the parent's request to outweigh this benefit.

If the therapy is not efficacious and potentially harmful, the clinician should discourage the parent from administering the intervention. The clinician may even be obligated to contact child protective services if the parent administering the intervention places the child at significant risk of serious harm. If the parent is requesting clinicians provide nonindicated life-sustaining measures, then the clinician can utilize a 7-step process for conflict resolution related to potentially inappropriate therapies, outlined in a policy statement from several professional societies.[36]

SUMMARY

SDM is a mainstay of clinical medicine, including pediatrics. The process of tailoring an SDM approach in pediatrics can be reached through 4 sequential questions.

1. Does the decision include more than 1 medically reasonable option (with only those that do have more than 1 option being within the domain of SDM)?
2. Does 1 option have a favorable medical benefit-burden ratio compared to other options (to determine if the decision will be clinician-guided or parent-guided)?
3. How preference-sensitive are the options to the parent?
4. What contextual factors are present that may tailor the type of SDM used?

The result of this process is to determine where a particular decision should lie on a spectrum from highly clinician-guided to highly parent-guided SDM.

Clinicians should also be mindful of how other decision-making models in pediatrics can be confused with SDM because of common communication strategies shared among them. Partnering with parents is still essential, even when they may decline all medically reasonable options or insist on therapies that do not appear to be medically reasonable. However, decision-making models other than SDM are necessary to adequately address these instances.

CLINICS CARE POINTS

- SDM should be utilized when there is more than 1 medically reasonable option.
- SDM in pediatrics exists on a continuum from clinician-guided to parent-guided. Which type is to be utilized depends on the medical benefit-burden ratio of the medically reasonable

options, how preference-sensitive the options are to the parents, and other contextual features.

- Collaborative communication techniques should be utilized in many models of decision-making; their use does not necessarily indicate that SDM is the appropriate decision-making model.
- Decision-making models other than SDM must be utilized to adequately address instances when parents decline all medically reasonable options or insist on therapies that do not appear to be medically reasonable.

DISCLOSURE

The authors have no relevant financial disclosures.

REFERENCES

1. Kon AA, Davidson JE, Morrison W, et al. Shared Decision Making in ICUs: An American College of Critical Care Medicine and American Thoracic Society Policy Statement. Crit Care Med 2016;44(1):188–201.
2. Ross FL. The philosophical underpinning of the family for pediatric decision-making. Pediatr Clin North Am, in press.
3. Seltzer RR and Thompson BS. Pediatrician as Advocate and Protector: An Approach to Medical Neglect for Children with Medical Complexity. Pediatr Clin North Am, in press.
4. Moon M. Duty to "Respect Autonomy" in the Pediatric Setting. Pediatr Clin North Am, in press.
5. Opel DJ. A 4-Step Framework for Shared Decision-making in Pediatrics. Pediatrics 2018;142(Suppl 3):S149–56.
6. Sawyer KE, Opel DJ. A stepwise framework for shared decision-making. In: Lantos JD, editor. The ethics of shared decision making. Oxford, Incorporated: Oxford University Press; 2021. p. 118–40.
7. Emanuel EJ, Emanuel LL. Four models of the physician-patient relationship. JAMA 1992;267(16):2221–6.
8. Whitney SN, Holmes-Rovner M, Brody H, et al. Beyond shared decision making: an expanded typology of medical decisions. Med Decis Making 2008;28(5):699–705.
9. Sandman L, Munthe C. Shared decision making, paternalism and patient choice. Health Care Anal 2010;18(1):60–84.
10. Muller-Engelmann M, Keller H, Donner-Banzhoff N, et al. Shared decision making in medicine: the influence of situational treatment factors. Patient Educ Counsel 2011;82(2):240–6.
11. Tilburt J. Shared decision making after MacIntyre. J Med Philos 2011;36(2):148–69.
12. Wirtz V, Cribb A, Barber N. Patient-doctor decision-making about treatment within the consultation—a critical analysis of models. Social science & medicine 2006;62(1):116–24.
13. Epstein RM, Peters E. Beyond information: exploring patients' preferences. JAMA 2009;302(2):195–7.
14. Whitney SN. A new model of medical decisions: exploring the limits of shared decision making. Med Decis Making 2003;23(4):275–80.

15. Murray E, Charles C, Gafni A. Shared decision-making in primary care: tailoring the Charles et al. model to fit the context of general practice. Patient Educ Counsel 2006;62(2):205–11.
16. Murray E, Pollack L, White M, et al. Clinical decision-making: Patients' preferences and experiences. Patient Educ Counsel 2007;65(2):189–96.
17. Kon AA. The shared decision-making continuum. JAMA 2010;304(8):903–4.
18. Gwyn R, Elwyn G. When is a shared decision not (quite) a shared decision? Negotiating preferences in a general practice encounter. Social science & medicine 1999;49(4):437–47.
19. Diekema DS. Parental refusals of medical treatment: the harm principle as threshold for state intervention. Theor Med Bioeth 2004;25(4):243–64.
20. Whitney SN, McGuire AL, McCullough LB. A typology of shared decision making, informed consent, and simple consent. Annals of internal medicine 2003; 140(1):54–9.
21. Elwyn G, Frosch D, Thomson R, et al. Shared decision making: a model for clinical practice. J Gen Intern Med 2012;27(10):1361–7.
22. Opel DJ, Vo HH, Dundas N, et al. Validation of a Process for Shared Decision-Making in Pediatrics. Acad Pediatr 2023. https://doi.org/10.1016/j.acap.2023. 01.007.
23. Hall v. Hilburn, 466 S. 2d 856 (Miss. 1985).
24. McCourt v. Abernathy, 457 S.E.2d 603 (S.C. 1995).
25. Johnston v. St. Francis Medical Center, Inc., No. 3-5, 236-CA, Oct. 31, 2001.
26. Institute of Medicine. Committee on standards for developing trustworthy clinical practice guidelines. Clinical practice guidelines we can trust. Washington, D.C.: National Academies Press; 2011.
27. Guyatt GH, Oxman AD, Vist GE, et al. GRADE: an emerging consensus on rating quality of evidence and strength of recommendations. BMJ Clin Res 2008; 336(7650):924–6.
28. American Academy of Pediatrics. Definitions explained: standards, recommendations, guidelines, and regulations. Secondary definitions explained: standards, recommendations, guidelines, and regulations 2017. Available at: https://www.aap.org/en-us/Documents/Definitions_StandardsGuidelines.pdf.
29. Bynum J, Passow H, Austin A, et al. Serious Illness and End-of-Life Treatments for Nurses Compared with the General Population. J Am Geriatr Soc 2019;67(8): 1582–9.
30. Periyakoil VS, Neri E, Fong A, et al. Do unto others: doctors' personal end-of-life resuscitation preferences and their attitudes toward advance directives. PLoS One 2014;9(5):e98246.
31. Morrow AM, Hayen A, Quine S, et al. A comparison of doctors', parents' and children's reports of health states and health-related quality of life in children with chronic conditions. Child Care Health Dev 2012;38(2):186–95.
32. Blumenthal-Barby JS, Krieger H. Cognitive biases and heuristics in medical decision making: a critical review using a systematic search strategy. Med Decis Making 2015;35(4):539–57.
33. Elwyn G, Frosch D, Rollnick S. Dual equipoise shared decision making: definitions for decision and behaviour support interventions. Implement Sci 2009;4:75.
34. Sherwin S. The politics of women's health: exploring agency and autonomy in health care. Philadelphia: Temple University Press; 1998.
35. President's commission for the Study of ethical Problems in medicine and biomedical behavioral Research. Making health care decisions: a report on the

ethical and legal implications of informed consent in the patient-practitioner relationship. Washington, D.C., 1982.

36. Bosslet GT, Pope TM, Rubenfeld GD, et al. An Official ATS/AACN/ACCP/ESICM/SCCM Policy Statement: Responding to Requests for Potentially Inappropriate Treatments in Intensive Care Units. Am J Respir Crit Care Med 2015;191(11): 1318–30.

Confidentiality in Primary Care Pediatrics

Mary A. Ott, MD, MA

KEYWORDS

- Adolescent • Confidentiality • Parent • Bioethics

KEY POINTS

- Confidentiality is an important practice because it recognizes the adolescent's emerging capacity, provides an opportunity for adolescents to take responsibility for their own health care, and facilitates the transition to adulthood.
- Confidentiality practices are in the best interest of the adolescent. Adolescents who are provided with confidential care and time alone with their physicians are more likely to disclose, to access needed care, and potentially have better health outcomes.
- Confidentiality addresses areas of great health inequities, and access to confidential care for sensitive topics such as sexual and reproductive health is considered a human right.
- Providers will need to be aware of system-level threats to confidentiality through electronic health records and online health portals.
- In contrast to assumptions, many parents support confidentiality practices and are willing to work collaboratively with their adolescent's pediatric provider.

INTRODUCTION

Confidentiality is a core component of adolescent primary care. However, it is also one of the most complex because pediatric providers must simultaneously recognize the emerging capacities of adolescents and navigate the evolving relationship between adolescents and their parents or caregivers. This article defines confidentiality, provides empiric and conceptual support for confidentiality, and offers practical advice on integrating confidentiality practices in the primary care of adolescents.

What Is Confidentiality?

A 14-year-old comes to clinic with a parent for a well-child check. You introduce yourself and set the expectation that part of the visit will be with both the parent and adolescent, part of the visit will be with the adolescent alone, and that certain types of information shared by the adolescent will be confidential. "What does that mean exactly?," the adolescent asks.

Indiana University School of Medicine, 410 West 10th Street, HS 1001, Indianapolis, IN 46202, USA
E-mail address: maott@iu.edu

Pediatr Clin N Am 71 (2024) 49–58
https://doi.org/10.1016/j.pcl.2023.08.002
0031-3955/24/© 2023 Elsevier Inc. All rights reserved.

In the context of adolescent health care, confidentiality has to do with flow of information among adolescents, parents or caregivers, and providers. When information is confidential, the adolescent controls the flow of information and must give permission for the information to be shared, even with parents or caregivers. When information is not confidential, parents and caregivers have access to the information. Confidentiality is related to, but differs from, consent. Consent is the process by which a competent individual is informed about treatment options and provides affirmative agreement to the proposed health-care plan. If an individual can consent to health care, they are entitled to confidentiality around that health care.

States have minor consent laws for safety and public health, recognizing that although it is generally desirable to involve parents and caregivers in adolescent health care, many adolescents will not access sensitive services such as family planning, sexually transmitted infection (STI) screening and treatment, or substance use treatment, if they are required to involve their parents or caregivers.[1] Because confidentiality is linked to health-care consent, the exact types of confidential information and services can vary from state to state. General medical information is usually not confidential, meaning that parents or caregivers have access to that information. Certain types of sensitive information will be confidential, meaning that you need the adolescents' permission to share with a parent or caregiver. Confidential information might include substance use, sexual behavior, STI screening, diagnosis and treatment, and contraception.[1]

At the physician level, confidentiality practices include time alone with the adolescent, discussing the range and limits of confidentiality, allowing adolescents to control the disclosure of sensitive information, and discussing situations where you would break confidentiality with the adolescent themselves before discussing with parents or caregivers. For pediatric practices and health-care institutions, confidentiality practices include having a policy for adolescent time alone with providers, identifying what information can be kept confidential, and ensuring electronic health access through visit summaries and portals support confidentiality. For governments, confidentiality practices include laws and policies that support adolescent confidentiality, and funding for confidential adolescent care.

How Are We Doing with Confidentiality?

The parent says that this is the first time confidentiality has been discussed with the adolescent, and the first time the parent has been asked to step out of the room.

Data suggest that we are not doing well with respect to providing adolescents with confidential care. In a nationally representative survey, only 42% of 15 to 17 year olds and 20% of 11 to 14 year olds reported time alone with their provider at their last preventive visit, and only 42% of 15 to 17 year olds and 24% of 11 to 14 year olds reported that their provider ever discussed confidentiality.[2] In that study, less than one-third of 14 to 17 year olds and fewer than 16% of 11 to 14 year olds reported discussion of any of the following sensitive topics: gender identity or orientation, safe dating, contraception, or STIs and human immunodeficiency virus (HIV).[2] Despite best practice recommendations,[3] few adolescents are actually receiving confidential care in the context of primary care.

Why Is Confidentiality Good for Adolescents?

The parent and adolescent want to know why time alone and confidential care? You reply that confidentiality is important component of keeping adolescents healthy and helping them transition to adulthood. Adolescents who receive confidential care learn to talk to a medical provider on their own and take more responsibility for their own health care. Confidentiality is a "safety valve" as confidential care provides the young person with another safe adult to confide in. Because confidentiality is a best practice in pediatrics, it is your office policy to provide confidential care to all adolescents.

The principle of beneficence strongly supports confidentiality. Public health data demonstrate that confidentiality practices and policies improve adolescent disclosure of risk behaviors, engagement in their own health care, access to sensitive services, and adolescent health outcomes. Research shows that adolescents provided with confidentiality assurances are more likely to disclose sensitive information, such as sexual behavior and substance use, to their providers.[4] Adolescents in primary care clinics who spent time alone with their provider, a best practice in confidential care, were more likely to think that they were a part of the health-care decision-making and were more engaged in their own care.[5] Conversely, when confidentiality is restricted, adolescents are less likely to access care, particularly care for sensitive topics, such as contraception. When faced with the possibility of parental notification for birth control, 40% of national sample of adolescents receiving care in family planning clinics would not access contraceptive care, instead relying on condoms alone or withdrawal; for those accessing care without their parents' knowledge, 70% would not access contraceptive care if providers were required to notify parents.[6]

The most important causes of adolescent morbidity and mortality—substance use, firearms and violence, suicide, unintended pregnancies and STIs/HIV—are all sensitive topics, with disclosure, access to care, and treatment directly influenced by confidentiality. In a nationally representative sample, teens whose providers spent time alone with them and communicated about confidentiality with the adolescent and parent were more likely to report discussions of sensitive topics such as gender identity, sexual orientation, sexual decision-making, STIs and HIV, and contraception.[2] Laws and policies that undermine confidential care also contribute to worsening access to services[6-11] and worse outcomes such as higher birth rates.[12-14]

What Does the Law Say?

The parent asks, "As the legal guardian, shouldn't I be the person to give consent and have access to my child's medical information?" You reply that there are also legal supports for adolescent confidentiality.

Legally, confidentiality is supported by a complex system of state health-care consent and confidentiality laws, federal statutes, and case law. The strongest legal support for minor consent is state law. Few states have laws that specifically address minor confidentiality; however, all states have some type of minor health-care consent laws, and when adolescents can consent to care, they should receive confidentiality around that care. Some of these laws describe groups of minors (<18 years in most states) who may consent for health care based on their status or are considered emancipated. These laws vary by state and may include married minors, minors serving active duty in the military, pregnant or parenting minors, minor heads of household, or minors who go before a judge and petition for emancipation. A second group of laws describe diagnoses and services for which minors may consent, and thus receive confidentiality. These laws vary state-to-state and may cover screening and treatment of STIs and HIV, contraception, abortion, prenatal and postpartum care, and substance use screening and treatment.[15] For example, as of this writing, all 50 states and the District of Columbia allow minors to consent to diagnosis and treatment of STIs; however, only 34 states have laws allowing minors to consent to contraception (**Box 1** for sources of updated information on your state). In the wake of the Dobbs decision, many states are passing laws that forbid minor access to evidence-based health care, such as recent state legislation restricting minor access to abortion and

---

Box 1
Resources on state policies

- Guttmacher Institute State Laws and Policies
  https://www.guttmacher.org/state-policy/explore/overview-minors-consent-law
- Power to Decide State Policy
  https://powertodecide.org/state-policy

American Academy of Pediatrics (AAP) State Advocacy
  https://www.aap.org/en/advocacy/state-advocacy/
  or stgov@aap.org

---

gender affirming care for minors.[1,16] Some states additionally require providers to notify parents or guardians when minors are provided with evidence-based health care, such as contraception. Pediatric providers will need to know their own state laws with respect to confidentiality, minor consent, and parental notification. Although national resources are available (see **Box 1**), the legal landscape is changing so quickly that pediatric providers may need to verify minor consent laws with their institutions.

Federal laws also support minor confidentiality, including strong protections for confidentiality around substance use disorder treatment, and the *Health Insurance Portability and Accountability Act* (HIPAA) *Privacy Rule*.[15] HIPAA not only allows confidentiality when care is protected by state law, but also allows confidentiality when the parent agrees and allows confidentiality in cases of provider discretion.[17] If medical care requiring confidentiality is not covered under state laws and the provider does not have an opportunity to discuss it with the parent, but a provider believes that confidentiality is in the adolescent's best interest, the provider may use their discretion, document their reasoning in the medical record, and provide confidential care. HIPAA protections can be maximized by practices that have an office policy on confidentiality that adolescents and parents are asked to review, and a provider who makes it a practice habit to discuss confidentiality with parents and adolescents at well visits and at visits for sensitive issues. For sexual and reproductive health, adolescents obtaining services at Title X funded family planning clinics are entitled to confidential care, and Medicaid regulations provide support for confidentiality in sexual and reproductive health because the regulations require states to provide confidential family planning services for all pregnancy capable individuals, which includes pregnancy capable minors.[15]

Do Adolescent Have the Developmentally Readiness for Confidential Care?

The parent expressed concern about their adolescent's readiness to access care without parental involvement. You gently point out that by 12 to 14 years of age, most adolescents can understand health information and apply it to their own situation. "But Doc," the parent says, "I *live* with a teenager, and I can tell you that they do not make decisions the same as you and I." The parent then cites incidences of risky behaviors and what the parent considered "poor" decisions on the part of the adolescent.

The principle of autonomy suggests that if a person has the capacity to make decisions about their health, we, as providers, should respect that decision-making. Health-care decision-making capacity includes the person's ability to understand the health information, appreciate how the decision would affect them personally, demonstrate logical thinking including weighing risks and benefits, and making a voluntary choice.[18] Health-care decision-making research using this framework suggests that adolescents demonstrate these abilities by 12 to 14 years of age.[19,20] These data show that adolescents given the space for confidential care will have the capacity to make decisions.

Yet the parent in the case is not wrong in their assessment of risk and that young people's decisions differ from adults. Adolescents have less decisional experience, and neuroscience research shows that adolescents are less risk adverse, have more difficulty with perspective taking, and have more difficulty in situations with emotion or distraction.[21,22] These data suggest that while pediatric providers should provide confidentiality, they also will need to provide decision-making support.

A Question of Human Rights?

The adolescent chimes in, "but don't I have a right to confidential care?" Human rights are seldom discussed in the United States, and when people refer to "rights," they are often referring to civil rights described in the US Constitution or in federal and state law. These civil rights are linked to US citizenship, or criteria laid out in the specific law. Human rights, in contrast, are rights that are inherent to all irrespective of citizenship, culture, gender, race, creed, or other characteristics, based on their shared humanity.[23] Human rights cannot be taken away. Outside of the United States, human rights have more salience. The right to the highest attainable health is considered a basic human right. In 2016, the United Nations Committee on the Rights of the Child delineated that an adolescents' right to the highest attainable health includes access to health education, information, and care for sensitive topics such as sexual and reproductive health that is adolescent-centered, equitable, free, and confidential.[24]

The general principles underlying adolescents' human rights include a positive and holistic approach to adolescent development, nondiscrimination, having policies and programs support adolescents' best interests, and the need for adolescents to be heard and to participate.[24] A human rights framework is particularly helpful for adolescent confidentiality because it is a developmental framework that not only includes progressive rights of the adolescent linked to their increasing capacity but also addresses evolving role of the parent. For adolescents, parents should shift from making decisions for the adolescent to providing the adolescent with the support and guidance needed to make their own health decisions. A human rights framework further obligates states to provide policies and programs that enable adolescents to actualize their human rights to health and to confidential care.

Confidentiality and Health Equity

Your pediatric practice serves a diverse but lower resource community. In a confidential interview, the adolescent discloses that their friend's sibling was shot. Their parents do not know that they were near the shooting because it was after their family curfew.

The health outcomes most influenced by confidential practices, including sexual and reproductive health outcomes, substance use disorder, violence (both perpetration and victimization) and mental health are health conditions where we see the greatest disparities in access to care and outcomes.[25,26] Black and Latino/a youth experience higher rates of STIs, rural youth experience higher rates of substance use disorder, and youth from high poverty areas experience higher rates of gun violence. Confidential care encourages disclosure, increases access to evidence-based care, and can potentially improve health outcomes.

Talking to Parents About Confidentiality

The parent believes that time alone is not a bad idea because they think that their child will be more likely to talk to you about sex, substance use, and other risk behaviors.

However, the parent is uncomfortable with the idea that parents themselves would not have access to the information that adolescent shares with you. The parent says, "I'm responsible for the teen and my health insurance is covering their care. If I don't have information about my child, I feel like I can't do my job as a parent."

In contrast to studies of adolescent perspectives on confidentiality, studies of parents and caregivers show complex perspectives on confidentiality and minor consent, with both positive and negative views. In a nationally representative survey of parents or guardians of 9 to 17 year olds, 24% believed time alone with providers was very important, and 42% believed time alone was somewhat important, with the remainder either neutral or opposed.[27] In a qualitative study in Texas, although some parents expressed misperceptions about anticipatory guidance including the idea that talking about contraception gives kids the message that they can have sex, other parents in this same group believed that pediatric providers played important roles in bringing up the conversation about sex, relationships, and contraception early.[28] In another qualitative study, Minnesota parents expressed that time alone sometimes came as a surprise, and that parents would handle time alone better if the parent had some earlier warning.[29] This speaks to the need to start confidentiality practices at a young age.

A sizable proportion of parents and caregivers want pediatric providers to talk to their adolescents about sensitive topics, even controversial ones. In a nationally representative study of parents of 15 to 17 year olds, 50% wanted the pediatric provider to talk to adolescents about sexual orientation, 58% gender identity, 71% safe dating, 79% contraception, and 89% STIs/HIV. In the same study, parents of 11 to 14 year olds differed only a small amount, with proportions ranging from 46% for sexual orientation to 82% for STIs and HIV.[2] Parent gender is important: In a 2007 survey of parents of 9 to 17 year olds, 66% of mothers but only 34% of fathers wanted their pediatric provider to discuss pregnancy prevention during well checks.[27]

Breaking Confidentiality and Navigating the Gray Areas

During your time alone with the adolescent, you inquire about substance use. They admit to using marijuana via an e-cigarette device 4 to 5 days per week. They note that they "feel better—much less stressed" when using marijuana, and believe that they are better able to relate to people and function in school. They note that many of their friends also use marijuana to "chill." Their grades are mostly B's, and they still participate in some after school activities. Their parent does not know, and they ask you to keep the information confidential, saying, "My parent would lose it if they found out."

The adolescent wants to know if you will break confidentiality. The two situations where pediatric providers must break confidentiality are when there is a threat to adolescent's life or the life of another person, or when the provider is legally mandated to report. This requires the pediatric provider to know the child abuse and mandated reporting laws in their state. When you discussed confidentiality with the adolescent, you let them know that confidentiality is not 100%, and that there can be situations where you, as their provider, will need to break confidentiality.

What this adolescent has disclosed is in a gray area. Frequent marijuana use is not an immediate threat to the adolescent or others, nor is there a legal mandate for you to report use. Yet it is clear that the adolescent would benefit from an intervention addressing their marijuana use, and the involvement of a parent or caregiver has the potential to help the adolescent. You also realize that your obligation is to the adolescent, that confidentiality is important for adolescents developmentally, and that breaking confidentiality without a strong reason sends a message that the adolescent cannot trust their pediatric provider. You opt to use a brief office-based motivational interviewing intervention, and arrange follow-up.

System-Level Threats to Confidentiality

At the end of the primary care visit, you would like to screen the adolescent for cardiovascular risk and for gonorrhea and chlamydia. In your time alone with the adolescent, you collect their personal cell phone number and let you know that the office will call with their STI test results. You mention to the parent that the office will call the parent with the lipid and hemoglobin A1c results. The parent says, "that won't be necessary — I have my child's portal login information and can check the laboratories myself in a day or so."

Increased patient access to the electronic health record (EHR), including automatic visit summaries, patient portals, and patient access to progress notes has given rise to a series of system-level threats to confidentiality. The *Affordable Care Act* required providers to give visit summaries or provide portal access.[30] The *21st Century Cures Act* requires that patients be able to have access not just to laboratory tests and diagnostic test results but also to outpatient progress notes.[31] Although these are important pieces of patient advocacy legislation, they present practical threats to adolescent confidentiality.

Patient portals can be a very positive component of adolescent primary care, with adolescents who have confidential portal access using their portals and reporting satisfaction with portal use.[32] However, portals also represent a threat to adolescent confidentiality. The story above is common. When parents and caregivers have full access to their adolescent's EHR portal, they can see confidential laboratory tests, medications, and provider notes. Because adolescent confidentiality protections are not always built into EHRs or into portal counseling and enrollment policies, the reality is that there are multiple points where confidentiality can be breached. In a quality improvement study in a large health system, 2307 out of 3701 (62%) adolescent portals were registered with a parent or caregiver email,[33] and in a study of parent/caregiver portal access in 3 children's hospitals, outbound messages were accessed by a parent/caregiver in 64% to 76% of portals.[34] Other examples include systems that do not have clear procedures for access to adolescent portals, to parents/caregivers asking their adolescents for login information for (often innocuous) reasons such as the parent/caregiver checking laboratories or making appointments.

Pediatric providers will need to be familiar with their EHR capabilities. Is there only a single access level to the entire EHR? Alternatively, is it possible to have 2 level access, where the adolescent can see the entire EHR and the parent has a more limited access that allows them to message providers and make appointments? Guidelines exist on adolescent EHR confidentiality protections,[31,35] and pediatric primary care offices and health-care systems will need to have policies on minor and parent/caregiver access.

SUMMARY AND CLINICS CARE POINTS

In summary, confidentiality is a series of practices that support the evolving capacity of the adolescent and assist parents and caregivers in shifting from making decisions for the adolescent to supporting the adolescent in making their own health decisions. For primary care providers, these practices include the following:

- Creating an office policy about confidentiality and making sure both adolescents and parents and caregivers are aware of the office policy.

- Starting confidentiality practices, such as time alone, early in adolescence, so both the adolescent and parent or caregiver are comfortable with confidentiality before the adolescent engages in risk behaviors.

- Within each visit, set expectations for confidentiality at the start of the visit with both the parent and adolescent together: "For adolescent visits, I have part of the visit with the parent and adolescent together, and part of the visit with the adolescent alone, bringing parents back at the end of the visit."

- Explain why you are providing confidential care. Explaining to parents and caregivers makes it clear that you all share the same goal, advancing the health and well-being of the adolescent. Reasons for confidential care include the following: (1) Improves adolescent safety, by providing another trusted adult for the adolescent to disclose to; (2) Helps the adolescent learn to talk to a health-care provider on their own; (3) Requires the adolescent to take responsibility for their own health care; and (4) It is your office policy and best practice.

- Let adolescents and parents/caregivers know what is confidential and what is not confidential. General health information, like lipid and diabetes screening, is not confidential, and providers can share this health information with parents or caregivers without asking the adolescent. However, certain sensitive information will be confidential, meaning that you need the adolescent's permission to share the information with parents.

- Explain when you will break confidentiality, including disclosure of something that is life threatening to the adolescent or another person, or something that you are legally mandated to report. Some providers give examples, such as an adolescent who is planning to kill themselves for harm to self, or an adolescent who has been raped as an example of mandated reporting. This practice can reassure parents. It also makes it possible for the provider to maintain their relationship with the adolescent even when the provider must break confidentiality. In this case, a provider might say, "Remember at the start of the visit when we talked about my breaking confidentiality if a young person tells me something that I legally have to report? Well, this is one of those situations."

- Reassure the adolescent and parent or caregiver that confidentiality does not equal secrecy. Although you, as the provider, will not disclose confidential information, you encourage adolescents to talk to trusted adults in their lives about sensitive issues because this allows adolescents to reflect on their own values and their family's values.

Although confidentiality practices can be a source of conflict between parents/caregivers and providers, they can also be a way for providers and parents or caregivers to support the adolescent in a healthy transition to adulthood.

DISCLOSURE

Dr Ott's spouse is an employee of Eli Lilly, Inc.

REFERENCES

1. Guttmacher Institute. An Overview of Consent to Reproductive Health Services by Young People. 2023 1 June 2023; Available at: https://www.guttmacher.org/state-policy/explore/overview-minors-consent-law Accessed July 1, 2023.
2. Sieving RE, McRee AL, Mehus C, et al. Sexual and Reproductive Health Discussions During Preventive Visits. Pediatrics 2021;148(2).
3. Hagan JF, Shaw JS, Duncan PM. Bright futures: guidelines for health supervision of infants, children, and adolescents. 4th Edition. Elk Grove Village, IL: American Academy of Pediatrics; 2017.
4. Ford CA, Millstein SG, Halpern-Felsher BL, et al. Influence of physician confidentiality assurances on adolescents' willingness to disclose information and seek future health care. A randomized controlled trial. JAMA 1997;278(12):1029–34.

5. Brown JD, Wissow LS. Discussion of sensitive health topics with youth during primary care visits: relationship to youth perceptions of care. J Adolesc Health 2009; 44(1):48–54.

6. Jones RK, Purcell A, Singh S, et al. Adolescents' reports of parental knowledge of adolescents' use of sexual health services and their reactions to mandated parental notification for prescription contraception. JAMA 2005;293(3):340–8.

7. Reddy DM, Fleming R, Swain C. Effect of mandatory parental notification on adolescent girls' use of sexual health care services. JAMA 2002;288(6):710–4.

8. Lehrer JA, Pantell R, Tebb K, et al. Forgone health care among U.S. adolescents: associations between risk characteristics and confidentiality concern. J Adolesc Health 2007;40(3):218–26.

9. Girma S, Paton D. Does parental consent for birth control affect underage pregnancy rates? The case of Texas. Demography 2013;50(6):2105–28.

10. Leichliter JS, Copen C, Dittus PJ. Confidentiality Issues and Use of Sexually Transmitted Disease Services Among Sexually Experienced Persons Aged 15-25 Years - United States, 2013-2015. MMWR Morb Mortal Wkly Rep 2017; 66(9):237–41.

11. Fuentes L, Ingerick M, Jones R, et al. Adolescents' and Young Adults' Reports of Barriers to Confidential Health Care and Receipt of Contraceptive Services. J Adolesc Health 2018;62(1):36–43.

12. Zavodny M. Fertility and parental consent for minors to receive contraceptives. Am J Public Health 2004;94(8):1347–51.

13. Guldi M. Fertility effects of abortion and birth control pill access for minors. Demography 2008;45(4):817–27.

14. Myers C, Ladd D. Did parental involvement laws grow teeth? The effects of state restrictions on minors' access to abortion. J Health Econ 2020;71:102302.

15. State Minor Consent Laws. A summary. 3rd Edition. NC: Center for Adolescent Health and the Law: Chapel Hill; 2010.

16. American Civil Liberties Union. Mapping Attacks on LGBTQ Rights in U.S. State Legislatures. 2023; Available at: https://www.aclu.org/legislative-attacks-on-lgbtq-rights Accessed 1 July, 2023.

17. English A, Ford CA. The HIPAA privacy rule and adolescents: legal questions and clinical challenges. Perspect Sex Reprod Health 2004;36(2):80–6.

18. Appelbaum PS. Clinical practice. Assessment of patients' competence to consent to treatment. N Engl J Med 2007;357(18):1834–40.

19. Grootens-Wiegers P, Hein IM, van den Broek JM, et al. Medical decision-making in children and adolescents: developmental and neuroscientific aspects. BMC Pediatr 2017;17(1):120.

20. Wilkinson TA, Meredith AH, Katz AJ, et al. Assessment of adolescent decision-making capacity for pharmacy access to hormonal contraception. Contraception 2023;110002.

21. Andrews JL, Ahmed SP, Blakemore SJ. Navigating the Social Environment in Adolescence: The Role of Social Brain Development. Biol Psychiatr 2021;89(2): 109–18.

22. Steinberg L. Does recent research on adolescent brain development inform the mature minor doctrine? J Med Philos 2013;38(3):256–67.

23. United Nations Office of the High Commissioner on Human Rights, What Are human Rights? 2023; Available at: https://www.ohchr.org/en/what-are-human-rights. Accessed July 1, 2023.

24. Office of the United Nations High Commissioner for Human Rights, Committee on the Rights of the Child. *General Comment on the Implementation of the Rights of the Child during Adolescence.* Geneva, Switzerland: United Nations; 2016.
25. Centers for Disease Control and Prevention. Fast Facts: Adolescent Health. 2023; Available at: https://www.cdc.gov/nchs/fastats/adolescent-health.htm. Accessed July 1, 2023.
26. Centers for Disease Control and Prevention. Mental Health: Poor Mental Health Impacts Adolescent Well-being. 2023; Available at: https://www.cdc.gov/healthyyouth/mental-health/index.htm#:~:text=Adolescent%20Mental%20Health%20Continues%20to%20Worsen&text=In%202021%2C%20more%20than%204,10%20(10%25)%20attempted%20suicide. Accessed July 1, 2023.
27. Dempsey AF, Singer DD, Clark SJ, et al. Adolescent preventive health care: what do parents want? J Pediatr 2009;155(5):689–694 e1.
28. Durante JC, Higashi RT, Lau M, et al. Parent Perspectives about Initiating Contraception Conversations with Adolescent Daughters. J Pediatr Adolesc Gynecol 2023;36(4):399–405.
29. Mehus CJ, Gewirtz O'Brien JR, Gower AL, et al. Opportunities to Improve Adolescent Sexual and Reproductive Health Services in Primary Care Clinics. Clin Pediatr (Phila) 2023;62(7):695–704.
30. Public Law 111–148, 2010 (124 Stat. 782) Patient Protection And Affordable Care Act Of 2010, US General Publishing Office. Available at: https://www.ssa.gov/OP_Home/comp2/F111-148.html. Accessed August 30, 2023.10.1016/j.ccc.2023.03.001
31. Carlson J, Goldstein R, Hoover K, et al. NASPAG/SAHM Statement: The 21st Century Cures Act and Adolescent Confidentiality. J Adolesc Health 2021;68(2):426–8.
32. Hagstrom J, Blease C, Haage B, et al. Views, Use, and Experiences of Web-Based Access to Pediatric Electronic Health Records for Children, Adolescents, and Parents: Scoping Review. J Med Internet Res 2022;24(11):e40328.
33. Xie J, McPherson T, Powell A, et al. Ensuring Adolescent Patient Portal Confidentiality in the Age of the Cures Act Final Rule. J Adolesc Health 2021;69(6):933–9.
34. Ip W, Yang S, Parker J, et al. Assessment of Prevalence of Adolescent Patient Portal Account Access by Guardians. JAMA Netw Open 2021;4(9):e2124733.
35. Pasternak RH, Alderman EM, English A. 21st Century Cures Act ONC Rule: Implications for Adolescent Care and Confidentiality Protections. Pediatrics 2023;151(Suppl 1).

Pediatrician as Advocate and Protector

An Approach to Medical Neglect for Children with Medical Complexity

Rebecca R. Seltzer, MD, MHS[a,b,c,]*, B. Simone Thompson, LCSW-C[d]

KEYWORDS

- Children with medical complexity • Child maltreatment • Medical neglect
- Advocacy • Clinical ethics

KEY POINTS

- Medical neglect, which can have profound impact on child health outcomes, is often difficult to diagnose.
- Children with medical complexity (CMC) are at greater risk for medical neglect due to complex, often cumbersome, medical care plans; medical fragility increasing risk if the medical plan is not followed; frequent health system engagement; and increased financial and psychosocial challenges.
- Although laws that require mandated reporting may make such requirements seem clear, the inherent nuance of medical neglect cases for CMC may make decisions (based in law, ethics, and clinical information) more complicated.
- Parental omission in the medical care of a child may be most compelling to medical providers, but resource and support availability and societal factors should also be considered.
- Medical neglect is a multifactorial problem that requires multifactorial solutions. Medical providers have a unique opportunity to partner with caregivers to identify barriers to care, provide support, and contribute to improved medical provision and care coordination for CMC, stronger caregiver–provider relationships, and better long-term health outcomes.

CASE PRESENTATION (PART 1)

"CJ" is a 12-year-old female with history of a rare genetic condition, multiple congenital anomalies, global developmental delay, spastic quadriplegia, and seizure disorder on

[a] Department of Pediatrics, Johns Hopkins School of Medicine; [b] Johns Hopkins Berman Institute of Bioethics; [c] Department of Population, Family, and Reproductive Health, Johns Hopkins Bloomberg School of Public Health; [d] Department of Pediatrics, Johns Hopkins Hospital
* Corresponding author. 200 North Wolfe Street, Room 2060, Baltimore, MD 21287.
E-mail address: Rseltze2@jhmi.edu

Pediatr Clin N Am 71 (2024) 59–70
https://doi.org/10.1016/j.pcl.2023.08.006

numerous medications. She receives continuous feeds via gastrostomy tube (GT) 22 hours per day and requires supplemental oxygen overnight. She uses a wheelchair and needs support with all activities of daily living. She lives at home with her Mom, Dad, and two younger brothers. When CJ was born, her Mom quit working to be her primary caretaker. Her Dad commutes to work 2 hours per day with the family's only car; he helps at home when he can but works long hours to make ends meet. They have no other family in the area. They qualify for overnight home nursing but have been unable to reliably secure nurses in their rural area. The family drives 90 minutes to see you at the nearest children's hospital-affiliated primary care clinic to maintain all of CJ's care within the same health system. CJ has seven specialists: gastroenterology, genetics, developmental pediatrics, ophthalmology, orthopedics, pulmonology, and neurology.

CJ has been a patient at your primary care clinic for the last 5 years and has done well overall with some occasional illness and rare hospitalizations for acute exacerbations of her chronic conditions. She presents to your clinic today with her mother and younger brothers for a well visit. On reviewing her chart, she has not been seen in your clinic since her last well visit 1 year ago and in the interim has missed several specialty appointments with genetics, developmental pediatrics, neurology, and gastroenterology/nutrition. She was last hospitalized for seizures 6 months ago after running out of medication. You review her growth chart and note that over the last year, she has lost weight and BMI has dropped from the 15th to second percentile. On examination, she looks thin, but otherwise well-appearing. She is sitting in her wheelchair, smiling with her Mom and brothers. Her GT site is clean and dry. The remainder of her skin examination is unremarkable without any signs of bruising, skin breakdown, or pressure wounds. Her neurologic examination and spasticity are at baseline and she seems comfortable. She has not had any seizures since resuming her medication during the last hospitalization.

As the primary care doctor, you are worried by her failure to thrive and that her parents did not seek care sooner with her noticeable change in body habitus. You are also concerned about the gaps in specialist medical care and the history of admission for seizures resulting from running out of medication. You question whether this meets criteria for medical neglect and are uncertain how to best advocate for CJ and her family.

BACKGROUND
Care Challenges for Children with Medical Complexity

Children with medical complexity (CMC), such as CJ, are patients with complex, chronic medical conditions with associated functional limitations, significant health care needs, and high health care utilization.[1] Their intensive daily care needs may include multiple medications with varying schedules or administration methods, multimodal therapies, and dependence on medical equipment or technology in the home (eg, ventilator, feeding tube, wheelchair). Families are tasked with navigating their child's care among a complicated and, typically, poorly coordinated network of medical providers, educational programs, and community or social services. In one study, caregivers reported spending numerous hours a week on care coordination (median 2 hours/week) and direct medical home care (11–20 hours/week).[2] In addition to challenges with care coordination and direct care delivery, studies show that families with CMC experience challenges with health care access (eg, insurance delays/denials, living long distances from specialty care), financial stress (eg, parent cutting back/quitting job to care for child, out-of-pocket medical expenses), and caregiver well-being (eg, burnout, impact on caregiver physical and mental health).[2,3] Medical complexity is shown to be a determinant of unmet health care needs, independent of race, ethnicity, language, insurance, or household income.[4]

What Is Medical Neglect?

Medical neglect occurs when a caregiver does not ensure necessary medical care (ie, caregiver fails to seek needed medical care for child or does not appropriately follow medical recommendations) resulting in harm or risk of significant harm to the child.[5,6] According to the American Academy of Pediatrics (AAP) clinical report on "Recognizing and Responding to Medical Neglect," there are several criteria that are necessary to make this diagnosis, including:[7]

1. A child is harmed or is at risk of harm because of lack of health care.
2. The recommended health care offers significant net benefit to the child.
3. The anticipated benefit of the treatment is significantly greater than its morbidity, so that reasonable caregivers would choose treatment over nontreatment.
4. It can be demonstrated that access to health care is available and not used.
5. The caregiver understands the medical advice given.[7]

There are various factors involving children, caregivers, physicians, health care systems, and the community that may contribute to a child not receiving needed medical care.[5–8] Any given situation is likely to involve multiple factors, interacting dynamically. Common issues include family financial stability, caregiver health, and mistrust of health care professionals; physician's ability to communicate clearly and coordinate a navigable plan of care; and local availability of specialty care and family support services. Medical complexity influences many of these factors and also introduces new variables to consider when approaching a case of potential medical neglect (**Table 1**).

Medical Neglect for Children with Medical Complexity

Children with disabilities are shown to be at higher risk for maltreatment. Based on a recent survey of child welfare agencies across the United States (unpublished data), medical neglect is considered the most common reason why CMC come to agency attention for both family support services and out-of-home placement. CMC are at greater risk for medical neglect for many reasons, including complex, often cumbersome, medical care plans; medical fragility increasing risk if the medical plan is not followed; frequent health system engagement; and increased financial and psychosocial challenges. Diagnosing medical neglect for CMC can be difficult, however, and teams may not consider the criteria noted above. In addition, medical care plans for CMC are at times based on provider preferences rather than evidence-based interventions that consider patient-specific risks and benefits. In fact, "data on effective therapies for CMC is often limited or non-existent."[8] If we cannot show that recommended health care offers net benefit substantially greater than the associated morbidity, a claim of medical neglect is questionable.

In cases where the possibility of medical neglect is unclear, it is important to work collaboratively with the family to identify barriers to care and ways to address them before labeling the case as medical neglect.[8] Even if it is determined that neglect has occurred, it is rare that the caregiver is solely responsible. Rather, CMC are cared for within a complex network of caregivers, professionals, services, systems, and policies that often share responsibility when a child's medical needs are not met.

Responding to Concern for Medical Neglect

Although specific language and regulations vary nationally, the federal government requires that all states have laws mandating medical professionals to report to child welfare authorities when they are concerned that a child has been maltreated. Studies reliably show, however, that pediatricians under-identify and underreport cases of

Table 1
Factors to consider for children with medical complexity and medical neglect[5-8]

	Factors to Consider
Child	Diagnoses, medical fragility Intensity of daily direct care needs Functional limitations, need for assistance with activities of daily living Technology/equipment use, risks of technology failure Medication/feeds/treatment regimen (complexity of care, timing, ease of adherence, risks of nonadherence) Attitudes and behaviors impacting care plan adherence Goals of care for child
Caregiver/family	Financial status and resources Family/friends as supports Other social supports Education level, health literacy Primary language Cultural and religious beliefs Caregiver physical/mental health, cognitive ability Trust in health care system/health professionals Caregiver burnout Family chaos, disorganization Access to transportation Employment (hours, pay, flexibility) Housing stability
Medical care team	Number of providers/types of specialists on care team Provider communication skills with patient/family; use of language access services (as appropriate) Provider–provider communication to ensure consistent care plan Access to case manager, care coordinator Availability of alternative communication methods (eg, text, e-mail, secure messaging) Availability and quality of home nursing (if eligible)
Health care system	Ease of scheduling appointments (clinic hours, specialists on same vs different days, direct contact for scheduling) Access to telemedicine vs in-person visits Insurance coverage, access to special needs coordinator
Community services	School-based services and supports (eg, IEP, 504 plan, school nursing) Social services resources (eg, TANF, SNAP, SSI, housing vouchers, and veteran's benefits) Access to respite services

Abbreviations: IEP, Individualized education plan; TANF, temporary assistance to needy families; SNAP, supplemental nutrition assistance program; SSI, supplemental security income.

maltreatment. Reviews indicate this is multifactorial, beginning with insufficient training to recognize signs of maltreatment, lack of clarity on what constitutes sufficient suspicion to report, negative past experience with child welfare, and misunderstanding regarding investigatory processes and outcomes.[9] In many cases, the primary reason for underreporting seemed related to fear that engaging child welfare authorities would undermine or destroy the provider's valued relationship with patients and families.[9] Additional research has shown that historical factors and implicit bias also impact rates of child welfare reporting, case acceptance, and child removal related to racial, ethnic, and socioeconomic inequities. Children of color are more likely to be evaluated and reported for maltreatment to child welfare authorities and are overrepresented in the foster care population. White children, matched on all other variables, are less likely to be considered for maltreatment assessment, to have a report made to child welfare, or to be investigated.[10]

In considering a child's medical needs and how those needs are met, the pediatrician should identify any modifiable factors that led to the concern for medical neglect (see **Table 1**), then collaborate with the family to address these factors while ensuring the child's safety and well-being. This may seem an overwhelming expectation, but is the most likely to meet the combined medical, family, and patient needs. The AAP outlines a continuum approach to responding to medical neglect concerns that progress from less to more restrictive interventions that address possible contributing factors.[7] This approach recommends starting with ensuring a shared language, through interpretation or translation (as needed) and active partnering with caregivers in sharing concerns and decision-making. If this is insufficient, providers are encouraged to then ensure adequate understanding, via counseling and education about the CMCs conditions, plan of care, and signs that warrant seeking medical care. Identification of additional caregivers, family supports, and community resources may further the caregivers' ability to meet the child's medical needs. Ensuring that the plan of care can be repeated by caregivers and clearly delineated in the medical chart, patient instructions, and discharge plans allows both medical providers and caregivers to reference those plans ongoing. When such endeavors are insufficient, increased contact with medical providers, using home visits, or partial hospitalization can be considered. This array of options is meant to reduce the likelihood of neglect or risk of harm to a child. If these less restrictive options are not available, efforts have been made but have been unsuccessful, or a child has been harmed, a report to the child welfare agency is indicated and should include the ongoing engagement and efforts that have occurred.[7]

Medical institutions may offer additional resources that assist in considering complex patient situations and assessment of maltreatment. Multidisciplinary child protection teams can help navigate these cases with input from specially trained medical providers and social workers. Ethics committee consults can also play a valuable role when the patient/family and health care team have conflicting opinions or goals regarding medical care plans.

For CMC, their very complexity may suggest additional strategies to improve care, such as increasing care coordination, simplifying medication and feeding plans in line with family schedule (as possible), and prioritizing tasks based on urgency. Not all aspects of a care plan may be equally important. For instance, the team may be able to help the family identify aspects that have greatest benefit or prevent the greatest harm. Further, some treatments, medications, procedures, or follow-up visits may not be essential and could be eliminated or paused for ease of care. In addition, families may be supported by linkage to local community and state-based resources specifically for children with special health care needs (eg, parent advocacy organizations, Title V programs, Medicaid waiver programs, equipment loan closets, and medical-legal partnerships). Finally, ensuring a child is enrolled in school and accessing eligible resources may support families and provide additional avenues for meeting a child's needs.

Children with Medical Complexity and Child Welfare Involvement

A family may engage the child welfare agency voluntarily to seek support or prevention resources or another individual (mandated reporter or otherwise) may contact authorities to report concern for maltreatment. When a caregiver has failed to ensure necessary medical care, either harming a child or indicating imminent serious harm, medical providers are mandated to report to the child welfare agency, even if the provider is working with the family to address potential underlying factors (see **Table 1**). Child welfare staff, if the case is accepted for investigation, must then determine if maltreatment occurred and if the child can remain in the family's care. Child welfare authorities may determine that the child may remain at home with specific services or supports in place or may petition for out-of-home placement via kinship care, foster care, or a congregate care setting.

Although data are limited, prior research shows that children with disabilities are more likely to have poor child welfare outcomes than their nondisabled peers; they are more likely to have a prolonged foster care course, unstable placements, and lower likelihood of permanency (ie, reunification with biological family or adoption).[11] There is a shortage of foster parents nationally, especially those willing and trained to care for a medically complex child. Significant delays in identifying an appropriate out-of-home placement are common for CMC, often resulting in prolonged hospital stays, well past medical readiness for discharge, or placement in congregate care rather than the preferred home-based care environment. In some circumstances, CMC require out-of-state placement when no appropriate resource can be identified locally. More data are needed to understand short- and long-term outcomes for CMC in foster care, including whether CMC placed in out-of-home care due to medical neglect actually demonstrate improved health and well-being outcomes.

ETHICS CASE APPROACH AND DISCUSSION

Ethical challenges arise in the clinical setting when multiple moral obligations are in conflict. Pediatricians regularly face ethical challenges in a variety of settings (eg, outpatient, emergency department [ED], inpatient, intensive care unit [ICU]) where concerns for neglect may arise. Approaching such cases through a thoughtful, ethics-guided lens can be limited by time constraints, clinical demands, and social factors. As a result, some clinicians may jump to suspecting neglect without seeking understanding of any case-specific contextual features.

Why Is This Case Ethically Challenging?

Much has been written about ethical challenges associated with reporting child maltreatment, especially in cases where there is not clear evidence of maltreatment. In trying to prevent harm to the child associated with medical neglect, how do we avoid introducing additional new harm while promoting well-being and maintaining a positive therapeutic relationship? Although laws that require mandated reporting may make such requirements seem clear, the inherent nuance of many neglect cases may make decisions (based in law, ethics, and clinical information) more complicated.

There are several relevant ethical principles to consider in this case.

- *Respect for autonomy:* Parents are given the legal responsibility to care for their child and the authority, within limits, to make decisions for their child that align with the family's values and priorities. There has been robust debate in the pediatric ethics literature about what threshold should be used for state entities (eg, child welfare, law enforcement, courts) to intervene in parental decision-making, such as when a parent refuses recommended treatment. Some rely on the "best interest standard," that a parent is obliged to make the decision that is in the child's best interest, whereas others argue that parents generally should be given wide latitude to make medical decisions for their child, as long as those decisions will not result in significant harm.
- *Nonmaleficence:* Pediatricians take an oath to "do no harm," but in complex cases, it may be difficult to prioritize which harms are to be avoided. In this case, multiple stakeholders might be guided by different values, including CJ, her parents, her

siblings, her primary care doctor, and her specialist medical providers. We must, therefore, consider what definition and whose viewpoint of harm to use.

- o *Narrow scope:* In a narrow medical view of harm, providers might only consider risks to CJ's health due to malnutrition, seizures, and missed medical follow-up. For CMC, gaps in care or poor adherence to medical plans may result in serious physical harm or even death. There are often times, however, that therapy and medications are of minimal benefit with identified side effects. In such cases, nonadherence may not indicate a net harm. Understanding how gaps in medical care specifically impact the child in question is the key to assessing risks of harm.
- o *Macro view:* Alternatively, providers may consider broader harms, beyond those specific to the child, such as trauma to the child and family via forced separation. In addition, damage to the therapeutic relationship may result in mistrust of the medical team and an increase in noncompliance with medical recommendations. Although some providers may consider foster care placement to be a medical intervention, there is variable quality and availability of medical foster care placements with limited to no data on outcomes for CMC served by the child welfare system. As such, there is no guarantee that removing CJ from her family will result in improved medical care and better long-term outcomes. She may have placement disruptions, as is common for CMC, resulting in more fragmented medical provision while in foster homes less versed in her specific needs.

- *Beneficence:* For CMC and their families, conversations about goals of care and quality of life can help establish what definition of "good" is being used by different stakeholders. Making medical care plans should be guided by these goals through a process of shared decision-making with the medical team and family. Ethical tensions can arise when medical treatments seen as the "optimal" standard of care for a medical condition conflict with the family's identified goals. For example, if the family's goal is to avoid discomfort, adhering to a frequent airway clearance regimen that is poorly tolerated by the child may conflict with that goal. When medical teams have difficulty navigating such conflict, palliative care may help the team reframe what should be considered "optimal" care, allowing for deviation from an identified or perceived standard.
- *Justice:* As suspicion for neglect is based on professional judgment, rather than specific, objective measures, there is risk to introduce bias. Prior studies show overreporting of minority and socioeconomically disadvantaged families and underreporting of white and socioeconomically advantaged families; it is important to be aware of this bias and strive for more equity in evaluation and reporting of maltreatment.[10] Structural inequities can also play a role in a family's access to resources and supports.

What Additional Information Is Needed to Guide Our Actions?

Jonsen and colleagues' four-topic method is a helpful tool to take a more comprehensive look at the relevant features of the case to help recognize where underlying ethical conflicts exist and how to navigate them in the clinical setting.[12] A more comprehensive look into case specifics including medical indications, patient/family preferences, quality of life and goals of care, and contextual factors may help. **Table 2** shows an example of the types of questions that CJ's pediatrician could consider in this case.

CASE PRESENTATION (PART 2)

After objectively outlining your concerns regarding CJ's weight and missed appointments to her Mom and Dad, who joined by phone from work, you ask them to share

Table 2
Applying the four-topic method to CJ's case

Medical indications
- What are the known serious risks of not adhering to the recommended plan of Care?
- Is CJ considered malnourished based on current growth parameters? Is it acute or chronic? What risks does she face due to her nutrition status?
- What are the potential causes of CJs poor weight gain?
  - Inadequate calories (eg, not receiving feeds as scheduled? feeding schedule not compatible with daily activities? overdue for feed adjustment? pausing feeds due to intolerance?)
  - Increased metabolic demand (eg, increased work of breathing? worsening spasticity? B symptoms?)
  - Increased output (diarrhea? vomiting?)
- Which specialty visits are essential and should be prioritized? Is there significant risk of harm from missing specialty visits?
- What medications does she currently take? What risks are there for missing any of these medications? Are all medications clearly effective/beneficial for CJ or could any be removed to simplify her regimen?

Contextual features
- What supports are in place for caregiving? (eg, help from family members/friends? home nursing? respite?)
- What is the family's current financial situation and how might that create a barrier to care?
- Does the child have adequate insurance?
- What additional supports/resources is the child/family eligible for?
- How does family's cultural/religious beliefs align with medical plan of care?
- What is family's primary language? Do they require interpretation/translation to understand spoken and written medical information?
- What is the family's preferred mode of learning (eg, visual, auditory, written, multimodal)?
- Do the parents have any physical or mental health diagnoses that impact their caregiving ability?
- Does the family have access to transportation to get to medical appointments and around the community?
- How do state laws (ie, mandated reporting) impact the case?

Quality of life
- How do the various treatments/medications impact quality of life, both positively and negatively, for CJ and family?
- How do the frequency of medical visits impact quality of life?
- Have goals of care been discussed with the family? Are medical care expectations aligned with goals of care?
- Any indication to involve palliative care in discussions about care plans?

Patient preferences
- Does CJ have any capacity to be involved in medical decision-making and medical care planning? If not, confirm who is authorized to serve as her proxy decision-maker. Typically, this is the biological parent(s), but always confirm.
- Do her parents have the capacity to understand the medical care plan and make decisions in the best interest of the child? Any limitations to decision-making capacity, such as substance use, cognitive impairment, and untreated mental health conditions?
- What is the threshold for state intervention in parental decision-making? Has it been met?

their concerns and thoughts. You learn that CJ started a new school 6 months ago that can accommodate her medical needs, but it is a 1-hour bus ride and feeds cannot be run during this commute. You communicate with the school and are told that feeds are restarted once she is settled in class, around 30 to 45 min after getting off bus. They also mention that feeds are sometimes paused during her school-based physical therapy (PT) and occupational therapy (OT). You calculate that she is likely getting 18 to 19 hours per day of feeds instead of the recommended 22 hours. The family is very happy with the school and the services she is receiving and thinks she is thriving in this new setting. They value this time she has around peers and they have noticed she seems happier returning to school after being home for 2.5 years due to COVID. She is also more active at school with PT and OT, which had been stopped when in virtual school. As the poor weight gain likely happened slowly over those 6 months, they state that they did not notice the change in her habitus. Now that you showed them the growth chart, they are appropriately concerned.

In regard to the missed specialty visits, you review the chart together and discover that although they had several no-shows, they attended 60% of their scheduled visits over the last 12 months. They plan to reschedule the others. Of note, during the visits that she attended it is clear that her weight was dropping over the last 6 months, but this was not mentioned to the family or noted in the assessment or plan of care. Per CJ's parents, there are several contributing factors to missed visits including (1) they only have access to one car and medical assistance transport has not been reliable in past, (2) their car is not modified to be wheelchair accessible, so it has become increasingly challenging to transport her to medical visits, (3) as CJ has grown, Mom has injured her back making lifting harder, (4) they did not want her to miss a lot of school as she was adjusting to the new setting and one visit usually requires missing a full day of school due to travel time.

In reviewing her medications, CJ's parents express frustration that she ran out of her seizure medications, in part because they were unable to contact the neurologist to request a refill, despite numerous calls to that office. They regret that they did not realize sooner she was out of refills. With 10 different medications and supplements, given multiple times per day, they sometimes have difficulty keeping track of when refills are needed.

What Actions Should We Take?

When considering what to do in this case, it is important to ask "what does this child need, and how can it best be provided?"[6] By using the AAP clinical report's "least to most restrictive" approach along with information gained using the four-topic method and speaking openly with relevant stakeholders (eg, parents, school staff, other providers), we can start to brainstorm action plans that maximally balance the ethical principles that are in conflict.

Objectively consider whether harm has occurred

As physicians, we are mandated to report to child welfare if there is concern that the child has been harmed or is at imminent risk of serious harm. In considering CJ's case, we must objectively consider whether this threshold to report has been met or whether less restrictive options are appropriate. There have been overt gaps in CJ's subspecialty care and she has lost weight. Overall, however, she appears well cared for, parents are seeking care when she is ill, and she is actively engaged in school and therapies. CJ's parents are open and engaged in discussing CJ's care needs and outline what steps they have made to ensure she is nurtured and healthy. Missed subspecialty appointments have not resulted in obvious harm to CJ. Although delays in refilling medication resulted in a hospitalization for seizures, the parents had attempted to contact the neurologist for refills and appropriately sought urgent medical care. Her weight loss, though concerning, did not require inpatient hospitalization, result in laboratory abnormalities, or impact her daily functioning. There had been no prior concern raised to the parents by other providers or school personnel regarding the weight loss. Given these considerations, CJ's presentation is not consistent with medical neglect that has resulted in reportable harm. There does not seem to be imminent risk of serious harm, though there are clearly risk factors that should be addressed to prevent worsening of her present condition. Based on this assessment, a child welfare report does not seem warranted at this time. Rather, the goal becomes collaboration toward addressing modifiable factors to decrease risk of harm.

Address modifiable risk factors

In CJ's case, there are clearly identifiable factors that contributed to her gaps in care and are modifiable. By addressing these factors, it is possible to avoid harm to CJ's health while maintaining the therapeutic relationship, respecting what matters most to the family, promoting quality of life, and supporting ease of caregiving. Some strategies could include.

- *Poor weight gain:* Working with CJ's gastroenterology and nutrition team, her parents, and school, create a feeding plan that provides necessary calories and is feasible within the known constraints. Once implementing a change in feeding plan, there should be regular check-ins with the medical team to ensure it is well tolerated and she is gaining weight as expected. Owing to transportation challenges, try to limit in person weight checks by scheduling tele-visit follow-ups, as possible. Inquire if weights can be gathered via the school nurse or as part of skilled nursing visits to the home.
- *Missed visits:* Work with family to prioritize essential medical visits—for example, (1) schedule visit with GI and nutrition ASAP to adjust feeds, (2) schedule overdue electroencephalogram (EEG) to monitor seizure control. To limit missed school days and transportation challenges, explore if multiple in-person specialty visits can occur on the same day. Connect family with resources that help fund accessibility modifications for vehicles.
- *Medication compliance:* Review medications with the family and identify possible opportunities to simplify medication regimen. Arrange for a skilled nurse visit to meet with the family at home to identify strategies to organize medications, make it easier to remember when medications are due and know when refills are needed. In creating a medication calendar, include the provider contact information to facilitate refill requests. Identify if an Internet application or computer interface may exist that may also serve this function. As the primary care doctor, suggest they contact you if they have difficulty obtaining refills from the prescribing specialist in the future. Explore availability of mail order medications with automatic refill requests sent to ordering providers.

Consider the role of medical providers and systems of care in the patient's medical situation

When CJ was losing weight and some of her medical needs were being neglected, who was responsible? Was it solely the responsibility of her parents who did not notice the weight loss or bring her to all appointments? How did the health care institution contribute by not having an agile system able to schedule multiple specialists on the same day, outside of school/work hours, or at satellite offices in rural areas? Did the neurologist's office or pharmacy contribute, by not having a better system for communicating about refills? Did the subspecialists who saw CJ over the past 6 months, but failed to comment on her poor weight gain, contribute to her neglect? When there is no means of reliable transportation or financial support for related costs (gas, tolls, parking), is there insurance or societal responsibility? The list can be endless. Although it is easier to blame parents when gaps in care occur, identifying the contributions of various stakeholders and systems increases understanding that medical neglect is a multifactorial problem that requires multifactorial solutions.

Although it is important to identify modifiable factors to address on the individual patient level, it is also important to recognize and advocate for system-level changes that would improve medical care for CMC more broadly.

By the time medical neglect becomes a concern, there have often been many missed opportunities to (1) recognize barriers that prevent a family from following a complex care plan, (2) adjust the care plan, and (3) put additional supports in place that may improve opportunity for success. In advocating for CMC and their families, pediatricians should recognize their critical role, beyond only as a mandated reporter, to be a mandated supporter. Perhaps then, providers and families can work together to decrease cases of medical neglect and the associated ethical challenges.

SUMMARY

When a child with medical complexity seems to be receiving substandard medical care and there is concern for medical neglect, it is often presumed that this is an overt failure on the part of the caregivers. Rather than only considering mandated reporting to child welfare in such instances, we encourage medical providers to consider their role as "mandated supporters." Consideration of contextual factors that may contribute to the patient's care, or lack of recommended care, may provide a wider vantage point for medical providers while contributing to a more patient- and family-centered approach to care. Understanding the lived experience of CMC and their caregivers, patient/family preferences, and quality of life through active dialogue and engagement in the medical plan of care may improve therapeutic relationships, medical care, and the patient's overall health. When child welfare authorities must be engaged, because efforts to remove barriers to care have failed, a child has been harmed, or the child is still at serious risk of harm, the agency and other stakeholders can be assured that the caregivers were engaged in establishing the care plan, understood and were prepared to implement it, and that available support resources had been engaged. The desire for all parties — patients, caregivers, medical providers, and child welfare — are aligned in ensuring the safety and medical needs of the child are met in the least intrusive manner possible.

DISCLOSURES

The authors have no conflicts of interest to disclose.

REFERENCES

1. Cohen E, Kuo DZ, Agrawal R, et al. Children with medical complexity: an emerging population for clinical and research initiatives. Pediatrics 2011; 127(3):529–38.
2. Kuo DZ, Cohen E, Agrawal R, et al. A national profile of caregiver challenges among more medically complex children with special health care needs. Arch Pediatr Adolesc Med 2011;165(11):1020–6.
3. Yu JA, Henderson C, Cook S, et al. Family Caregivers of Children With Medical Complexity: Health-Related Quality of Life and Experiences of Care Coordination. Academic pediatrics 2020;20(8):1116–23.
4. Kuo DZ, Goudie A, Cohen E, et al. Inequities in health care needs for children with medical complexity. Health affairs 2014;33(12):2190–8.
5. Boos SC, Fortin K. Medical neglect. Pediatr Ann 2014;43(11):e253–9.
6. Stirling J. Understanding Medical Neglect: When Needed Care Is Delayed or Refused. J Child Adolesc Trauma 2020;13(3):271–6.

7. Jenny C, AAP Committee on Child Abuse and Neglect. Recognizing and responding to medical neglect. Pediatrics 2007;120(6):1385–9.

8. Coller RJ, Komatz K. Children with Medical Complexity and Neglect: Attention Needed. J Child Adolesc Trauma 2020;13(3):293–8.

9. Jones R, Flaherty EG, Binns HJ, et al. Clinicians' description of factors influencing their reporting of suspected child abuse: report of the Child Abuse Reporting Experience Study Research Group. Pediatrics 2008;122(2):259–66.

10. Lane WG, Seltzer RR. How Should Clinicians and Health Care Organizations Promote Equity in Child Abuse and Neglect Suspicion, Evaluation, and Reporting? AMA J Ethics 2023;25(2):E133–40.

11. Seltzer RR, Johnson SB, Minkovitz CS. Medical complexity and placement outcomes for children in foster care. Child Youth Serv Rev 2017;83:285–93.

12. Jonsen AR, Siegler M, Winslade WJ. Clinical ethics: a practical approach to ethical decisions in medicine. 6th edition. New York, NY: McGraw-Hill; 2006.

Establishing Goals of Care in Serious and Complex Pediatric Illness

Carrie M. Henderson, MD[a], Renee D. Boss, MD, MHS[b],*

KEYWORDS

- Goals of care • Pediatric complex care • Chronic critical illness • Palliative care

KEY POINTS

- Creating cohesive goals of care in complex pediatric illness may be threatened by a misaligned understanding of a family's values and desires.
- Cohesive goals of care require attention to team unity regarding prognosis, in-depth exploration of family context, and consistent communication.
- Blended goals of care may help families and clinicians align different viewpoints about the best course of action.

INTRODUCTION

An increasing number of children are living for months and years with enduring medical conditions that have substantial impact on their functioning and longevity. Several definitions are used to describe this population. The cohort of children with "medical complexity" are those with chronic health problems that result in functional limitations and intensive use of health services and resources.[1,2] Children with "chronic critical illness" have repeated and prolonged hospitalizations and multiple chronic medical technologies.[3] Children with "serious illness" have a high risk of death in childhood.[4] Taken together, these definitions delineate patients with varying levels of long-term prognostic uncertainty, intensive interactions with medical systems, functional limitations, and often home medical technologies that shape the child's and family's quality of life. This article will use the shorthand "children with serious/complex illness" to denote this group of patients.

[a] Department of Pediatrics, Center for Bioethics and Medical Humanities, University of Mississippi Medical Center, 2500 North State Street, Jackson, MS 39216, USA; [b] Department of Pediatrics, Johns Hopkins School of Medicine, Johns Hopkins Berman Institute of Bioethics, 200 North Wolfe Street, Suite 2019, Baltimore, MD 21287, USA
* Corresponding author. Department of Pediatrics, Johns Hopkins School of Medicine, Johns Hopkins Berman Institute of Bioethics, 200 North Wolfe Street, Suite 2019, Baltimore, MD 21287.
E-mail addresses: rboss1@jhmi.edu; Rboss1@jh.edu

Pediatr Clin N Am 71 (2024) 71–82
https://doi.org/10.1016/j.pcl.2023.08.008
0031-3955/24/© 2023 Elsevier Inc. All rights reserved.

Data suggest that such children account for at least one-third to one-half of patients in US general pediatric wards[5] and neonatal (NICU)[6] and pediatric intensive care units (PICU).[7] They are also the primary utilizers of multidisciplinary pediatric outpatient services, including subspecialty providers, home nursing, occupational and physical therapies, and medical equipment providers.[8] Some of these interactions with health care providers reflect decision points: *Should a new medication be added for a distressing symptom? Is a risky surgery warranted, given declining quality of life? Should home respiratory support be intensified? Or stopped? What are the options when a family's daily care needs outstrip their community supports? How do we transition a child to adult services? When is it the right time to consider advance directives?* For children with serious/complex illness, the answers to these decisions rarely derive from a strong evidence base and often depend heavily on the family's goals of care (and by "family" we include those with central roles in a child's life and decision-making, eg, parents, extended relatives, guardians, etc.).

In their systematic review, Secunda and colleagues[9] offer an operational definition of goals of care that includes (1) what is hoped to be achieved overall for a child's care/condition, (2) grounding in both the immediate and big picture clinical course, (3) what is most important to the patient/family, and (4) a focus on how the decision at hand is impacted by these reflections on overall prognosis, clinical logistics, and values. The authors note that the essential benefit of setting intentional goals of care is to support families, to ensure that they have a role in decision-making, and so that patients do not receive less or more care than is desired.

Despite the importance of setting, communicating, and revisiting goals of care for children with serious/complex illness, multiple studies suggest that this process breaks down. Using a sample case for illustrative purposes, this article will explore common challenges to cohesive goals of care in complex pediatric illness: prognostic uncertainty, diffusion of medical responsibility, individual family context, and blended goals of care.

PROGNOSTIC UNCERTAINTY

Case: "Soraya Greene" had an uncomplicated infancy. At 18 months, she stopped gaining weight, coughed with feeds, said no words, and stopped walking. Subspecialty evaluation was delayed by transportation barriers and insurance gaps, so at 22 months Soraya was admitted for multidisciplinary work-up. During a 6 week hospitalization, her parents received the diagnosis: Soraya has a degenerative neurologic condition without cure. Among patients with this condition, the prognosis is variable: death in early childhood, slow progression with survival to young adulthood, and rare long-term survival are all possible. Progressive difficulty with feeding and breathing are likely.

The parents initially doubted the diagnosis and only intermittently attended subspecialty outpatient visits. When Soraya reached 3 years, the neurologist called the pediatrician with worries about disease progression. "I cannot be sure what her course will be," the neurologist said, "but if the family wants to prolong her life with medical interventions, we need to prepare for those decisions." The pediatrician meets with the parents to discuss goals of care and, if they are amenable, an advance directive. Soraya's parents say they want whatever it takes to give Soraya a "good quality of life" but don't want her to have "unnecessary suffering."

Clinical Questions
- How is "good quality of life" determined?
- How is "suffering" determined?

• What is intersection between pediatric goals of care and advance directives?

With advances in diagnostic and therapeutic tools, clinicians are increasingly able to put a name to a child's medical condition and to treat or at least ameliorate that condition. Yet prognostic uncertainty may only increase: *Will a novel treatment make the child's daily life better or worse? Will interventions prolong life? Will a plan of care allow a child to go home, or will they become dependent on inpatient care?* Some parents find prognostic uncertainty liberating: it allows hope that the child will exceed expectations. Families of infants recently diagnosed with serious/complex illness, for example, are more likely to opt for tracheostomy/home ventilation than are families of older children who have been living with similar conditions, because families of infants are more optimistic about clinical improvement.[10] Other families find prognostic uncertainty extremely burdensome, as demonstrated by Aite and colleagues[11] who showed that lower-mortality fetal conditions with widely variable outcomes were more anxiety-provoking to pregnant women than higher-mortality fetal conditions with a predictable outcome. Clinicians also have different reactions to prognostic uncertainty, with risk of being overly pessimistic[12] or overly optimistic.[13] In Soraya's case, the prognosis for her serious/complex illness is uncertain, but a shortened lifespan is likely. Her parents are already thinking about her quality of life and potential suffering.

"Quality of life" is a term that first showed up in the medical literature in the 1960s.[14] A proliferation of quality-of-life definitions and measures have been proposed since then, typically including the domains of physical, mental, and social functioning. Quality of life is generally in the eye of the beholder, meaning individuals with similar states of functioning may rate their quality of life differently. An individual's perception of a "good" or "acceptable" quality of life may also expand as the person adjusts to evolving functional status.

Assessing quality of life in children of varying developmental stages and abilities is especially complicated. Children with serious/complex illness may not be able to directly report their experiences of comfort, contentment, pain, relationships, etc. Often we rely on family report, which may conflate child and family experience. For instance, a mother and father of a child with serious/complex illnesses may rate the child's quality of life differently based on the parent's own role in the child's daily care. Adding to the intricacy of gauging a child's quality of life are the multiple studies showing that pediatric health care providers tend to rate a child's quality of life lower than families do,[15,16] especially for patients with neurologic impairment.[17] Given these factors, clinicians should generally defer to family assessment of an acceptable quality of life for a child who cannot contribute to the discussion. For Soraya's family, the next questions the pediatrician could ask might be, "*What does a good quality of life look like for your daughter?*" and "*What would an unacceptable quality of life look like?*"

Like quality of life, "suffering" is a concept that is often central to decision-making for children with serious/complex illness, yet equally vexing to define and assess. Core elements of suffering are generally physical and/or mental pain and distress. As with quality of life, the assessment of a child's suffering can be hard to disentangle from the experience of family. A parent may feel intense distress when their child has seizures, for example, but it is hard to know what the child is experiencing. The concept of "unnecessary suffering" that Soraya's parents raise with their pediatrician suggests they may find some degree of suffering acceptable to attain a goal. Some families may accept their child's discomfort with a tracheostomy, for example, if it means the child can be home with and a part of the family. There is no clear-cut threshold at which a child's suffering is so severe that irrevocable acts, like withholding or withdrawing life-sustaining therapies, should be considered. The risk for health care provider bias is real, when provider perceptions of a child's suffering might actually reflect personal values that the child's life is not worth living.[18] There are notable cases where clinician assessment of a child's suffering led them to seek to override the parent's assessment,[19] and ethical and/or legal consultation can be helpful in extreme cases. Absent such concerns, clinicians should defer to the family assessment of suffering when a child cannot contribute to the discussion. For Soraya's family, the clinician could ask *"What do you think would be some signs that would tell us that Soraya is suffering?"*

Soraya's parents covey that their goals of care include a "good quality of life" and avoiding "unnecessary suffering." The clinicians want to help them consider how these goals map onto decisions about medical care, including life-sustaining therapies. Nonurgent discussions of these topics, when a child is not in a medical crisis, may feel uncomfortable for clinicians who worry about frightening or distressing patients and families.[20] Multiple studies show low rates of pediatric advance directives, even among children with the most serious/chronic illnesses.[21] A formal advance directive may be less critical for pediatric versus adult patients, since parents are usually the legal decision-makers and are usually present to make medical decisions. It is important to note the multiple studies showing that many parents are open to discussions about life-sustaining therapies, perhaps particularly when they are worried that the treating medical team won't really know their child.[20–22] For children with serious/complex illness who have multiple hospitalizations and dozens of involved clinicians, there is a real risk that the clinicians managing a medical crisis will not be fully aware of the child's complex history. Importantly for the pediatrician, families prefer having conversations about advance directives in the context of a longitudinal relationship.[23]

In sum, intentional and timely conversations with families are the first step in establishing goals of care in situations with prognostic uncertainty. These conversations can build trust with families, even when the topics are emotionally difficult. Clinicians can guard against inserting their own values into these discussions by helping the family articulate their definitions of an acceptable and unacceptable quality of life.

DIFFUSION OF RESPONSIBILITY

Case, continued: Soraya presents to the emergency department 6 months later with an aspiration pneumonia and is intubated for acute respiratory failure. Her labs and imaging show evidence of chronic respiratory insufficiency and neurologic progression of her disease rendering her airway protection mechanisms dysfunctional. She has difficulty separating from the ventilator. During a long PICU stay, this new group of physicians directing her care recommend surgical interventions to mitigate ongoing risk of respiratory failure and acute illness: a gastric feeding tube (G tube), a tracheostomy (trach), and a ventilator for home. Pulmonary physicians are involved as well as the neurology team; prognostic uncertainty persists. The family has not shared with this new team the details of the recent goals of care discussion had with the primary pediatrician; the family is confused by the recommendations of the new team.

Clinical Questions
- How do acute care hospital processes impact the goals of care for children with serious/complex illness?
- What strategies exist for closing gaps in inpatient/outpatient care coordination?

Diffusion of responsibility in clinical care is a long-recognized phenomenon wherein organ- or disease-based teams operate in individual silos with little interteam communication about a child's overall prognosis. Rooted in the psychological phenomenon of the bystander effect,[24] multiple stakeholders focus on their own disease or organ system, believing someone else is taking on the mantle of responsibility, ultimately leaving no one in charge.[25] In ICU systems, rotating critical care physicians may act as the "team leader" to coordinate with various subspecialists and team members, but this has its difficulties as well. ICU physicians are trained to react to acute problems, not chronic care coordination, and ICU training programs focus more on technical skills than communication. The moving parts of a busy ICU dictate frequent attending turnover with handoffs of information targeted to urgent problems. Large interdisciplinary teams with multiple learner levels try to coordinate the flow the information between all of the subspecialty teams and the family.[26]

The limitations of these processes likely have the greatest impact on the growing group of children with serious/complex illness who often spend time in an ICU.[27] These patients require extensive care coordination, broadly defined as a family-centered, assessment-driven, and team-based activity that addresses the comprehensive needs of families.[28] In the context of large and siloed medical teams, care coordination between them is key to ensuring that interventions are both medically beneficial and in line with the family's goals. Without an intentional approach to team care coordination, families are left to filter and interpret conflicting information and to bridge communication gaps between care teams. In many institutions, this has led to the rise of inpatient/outpatient pediatric hospitalist and complex care teams to serve as the "quarterbacks" for children with serious/complex illness, filling the growing deficits between the pediatric health care system, and the historic surge in childhood morbidity and chronic disease.[29] Across the country, the growth of complex care teams has worked to promote care coordination and alleviate fragmentation and gaps, especially as the child goes from outpatient to inpatient and back home again.

Complex care teams may or may not serve as an outpatient medical home; when they do not, as in Soraya's case, the outpatient pediatrician may still be excluded from contributing to goals of care discussions in the hospital. Because inpatient medical care for children with serious/complex illness is often centralized to academic and/or large hospitals,[7] families like Soraya's may rely heavily on local pediatricians. For Soraya, who is experiencing an acute-on-chronic decline, her pediatrician holds unique perspective about her life up to now, her family's wishes and home life context, and a more comprehensive view of her gradual decline. Families of children who require frequent hospitalization clearly value their primary pediatrician's input when they are hospitalized, stating it improves interdisciplinary coordination and aids in decision-making.[30] Invitations to planned care conferences or family meetings, weekly phone calls for updates or check-ins, and web-based face-to-face participation in rounds or meetings are ways to include a primary care provider in creating goals of care.

It should be noted that, even when a reasonable degree of care coordination exists for children with serious/complex illness, clinicians may still struggle with a team-based approach to medical decision-making. A survey of NICU and PICU providers about professional responsibility for consensus decision-making noted that most providers did not feel a responsibility to achieve consensus, although most stated they would try for consensus around a high-stakes intervention for a child.[31] Most also agreed that conflicting recommendations about an intervention should be disclosed to a family. The literature reveals descriptions of a few team decision-making processes for children with serious/complex illness,[32] but this is an area that must clearly expand to meet the needs of this growing population.

In sum, the majority of children with serious/complex illness are cared for by large numbers of clinicians in the inpatient and outpatient setting. When these clinicians act in silos rather than as a coordinated team, families can become confused by disparate information and recommendations. The goals of care for a child will become fragmented without intentional processes for team coordination.

INDIVIDUAL FAMILY CONTEXT

Case, continued: During her PICU admission, Soraya's parents consider how their social circumstances relate to the home medical technologies (g-tube, tracheostomy, home ventilator) the doctors are recommending. The parents have limited transportation and are stressed about living several hours away from any pediatric hospital. They worry about the impact of bringing medical technology and home nursing into their home, and how it might affect their other children. In their interactions with the clinical team, they want to appear to be agreeable to "do what Soraya needs" but privately they wonder if it would be wrong to not pursue home medical technology and allow Soraya to die naturally.

Clinical Questions
- How does individual family context impact medical decisions for children with serious/complex illness?
- What strategies exist for preventing bias when considering family context?

Family context relevant to a child's well-being includes many elements of home and community: housing adequacy, transportation, financial vulnerability, parent physical and mental health, sibling needs, degree of extended family supports, access to community resources, childcare options, school resources, local respite, etc. For children with serious/complex illness, medical needs often place growing stressors on family context. A stressed family context, in turn, will have impact on a child's medical care and medical outcomes.[33]

Family life can be profoundly impacted by pediatric home medical technology.[34,35] Home ventilation via a tracheostomy, along with feeding per surgical gastric tube, requires some of the most complex home care because 24/7 assessment, monitoring, and intervention is needed. Historically, mechanical ventilation was only provided in an ICU setting but advances in equipment development and tracheostomy care enable children to receive this technology in a home setting. Parents become responsible for a level of care otherwise delivered by highly trained clinicians in a hospital; the rate of adverse events with home ventilation is significant.[36,37] Despite the training that families get to manage medical equipment, recent data suggest families feel unprepared for the enormous effect of home ventilation on their day-to-day lives. They report significant stress on their relationships, employment, financial security, and personal well-being—most families report these factors were not emphasized during the decision-making process about home medical technology.[34,38] The impact of home ventilation also shapes the child's life in a variety of ways: limitations to travel and mobility, hindering some aspects of development, continued infections or complications, and isolation due to medical fragility.[39] Most families who choose home ventilation report that they would make the same decision again, but also admit to significant challenges and burdens that were not discussed or anticipated.[34,40]

Establishing goals of care regarding treatments or interventions with broad impact on home life should intentionally explore social realities and expectations.[32] This might include discussing that one parent may need to stop working, or the family might need to buy a different vehicle, or may have limited home nursing, or may even want to relocate to a community with more resources. All of these factors could impact family stability, which impacts home care, which impacts child health outcomes.

Fairness and justice are important considerations: only addressing family context for some families of children with serious/complex illness risks bias. A standardized approach to including family context in serious decision-making is one way to protect against that bias. Palliative care engagement, with their philosophy and orientation toward family-centered decision-making, can be helpful. Palliative care providers also bring skills in considering alternatives to life-sustaining treatments and interventions, as Soraya's family wonders what it might look like if they decline the physicians' recommendation for medical technology. Ethics consultants may also be helpful in weighing risks and benefits of pediatric interventions with respect to a family's unique context. Families should be encouraged to reach out to other experienced parents, perhaps via online groups, to learn more about what life might be like if they choose, or decline, a particular medical intervention for their child.[41,42]

In sum, family context is an important consideration in medical decisions with broad impact on home life. When family context is not explored, we risk leaving families unprepared, undermining family stability and child medical outcomes. Systematic, skilled evaluations can reduce bias in determining how family context maps onto medical decisions.

BLENDED GOALS OF CARE

Case, continued: Soraya's parents feel she is still fighting and are not ready to fully shift to end-of-life care. However, they have decided that home medical technology is not right for Soraya or their family. The family wants to take Soraya home on her medicines and nasal cannula, and to continue feeding her by mouth, understanding this approach will leave Soraya susceptible to aspiration and lung infections. The inpatient provider teams worry Soraya will have poor nutrition, increased infections, and hypoxia. Her outpatient pediatrician has concerns about accepting professional liability for Soraya's well-being once she is home, given unclear parameters for growth and vital signs. The family is offered home hospice but is not ready to enroll. They would like to avoid, though have not ruled out, further hospitalizations as Soraya's health declines.

Clinical Questions
- What are blended goals of care?
- How can clinicians support families who have blended goals of care?

Pediatric medical decision-making is often based in the best interest standard wherein clinicians and families come together to create plans of care that best serve the child's health interests. Clinicians typically establish the scientific guardrails defining which treatment options are entirely beneficial to the child and therefore "obligatory" (eg, the parents cannot be allowed to refuse), and which treatment options are entirely without benefit and therefore "unacceptable" (eg, the parents cannot be allowed to elect them). These scientific guardrails delineating benefit and harm are generally based on clinical evidence regarding pediatric populations without serious/complex illness. Substantial ambiguity characterizes which treatment options might help or harm a child with a progressive illness and limited lifespan. If Soraya goes home with a nasal cannula and oral feeding, she may die sooner, but the time she has can be focused on comfort and family. If she receives a tracheostomy and g-tube, she might live longer (though not necessarily), but the extra time she has might be lived in the hospital, away from her family. Neither option is without potential benefit or harm, so it is difficult to consider either option "obligatory."

Some ethicists advocate for the "zone of parental discretion," suggesting that parents have ultimate decisional authority about the plan of care for their child even when clinicians feel the parents' plan is suboptimal.[43,44] Many families of children with serious/complex illness reject singular goals of care, opting for some blend of life prolongation and life enrichment. "Blended" goals of care often translate into a trial of, or limited use of, therapies with potential to reverse or slow a child's decline, with a priority for withholding/withdrawing those therapies that reduce the child's quality of life.[45] The process of forming blended goals of care varies with individual circumstances. Blended goals may be the result of a compromise when families seek one treatment path but clinicians recommend another. Blended goals may be derived for one specific treatment scenario, for example, a child's acute pneumonia, or they may describe the global approach to that child's care. Blended goals may limit one very burdensome intervention even as they escalate multiple, less burdensome interventions. Finally, blended goals may evolve by default, for example, simply because some treatments are tried and others are not, or they may be intentional goals set to direct a child's care. Blended goals are often a progressive series of compromises that aim to match family's values regarding their child's care. Blended goals avoid the "do everything versus do nothing" dichotomy and respect parents' wisdom regarding their child's experiences of their medical care.[46]

Clinician–family disagreement about Soraya's care likely reflects different perspectives regarding the desired outcome for Soraya. The clinicians are prioritizing best practice standards with a goal of sustained periods of health and longevity of life. The parents appear to be situated in the gray zone between palliative and curative intent. Their blended goals to orally feed Soraya and go home with nasal cannula, while accepting future hospitalizations for antibiotics and supportive care, create unease among inpatient and outpatient clinicians who wonder about their medical, legal, and ethical responsibilities to the child. Hospice engagement is one way to align clinician–family goals and create an outpatient, individualized treatment plan that is family-centric and medico-legally straightforward. This option is increasingly available and flexible with the rise in insurance coverage for concurrent care, for example, simultaneous curative and hospice services.[47]

In situations where home hospice is not involved, inpatient and outpatient clinicians must decide how to accommodate blended goals of care for children with serious/complex illness. Palliative care teams may offer support, given their expertise in managing children of all ages and diagnoses who are approaching end of life. They may be able to make recommendations regarding what vital signs parameters and nutrition goals could bridge the gap between what is achievable at home and what will optimize the child's well-being. Clear documentation about why nonstandard clinical parameters are being followed, and what those parameters are, will promote consistency between team members. Clinicians should also clearly communicate to families, and document, any potential risk of blended goals. In Soraya's case, if clinicians accept the parents' goal of minimal home respiratory support (nasal cannula), the parents should know that low oxygen can injure Soraya's brain and body, making future hospital interventions less likely to work. Finally, where clinicians cannot come to agreement about blended care goals, ethics consultation is recommended.

Although most decision-making models have a clear beginning and end, decisions for children with serious/complex illness resemble an evolving process without discrete boundaries.[48] Many families of children with serious/complex illness do not have dichotomized care goals of prolonging life versus comfort care. Instead, families often have iterative goals that are blended, that is, some medical interventions to extend life but not at the expense of quality of life. Clinicians can engage palliative care, hospice, and ethics resources to help them support families in developing blended goals of care.

SUMMARY

An increasing number of children are living for months and years with serious/complex illness that includes long-term prognostic uncertainty, intensive interactions with medical systems, functional limitations, and often chronic medical technologies that shape the child's and family's quality of life. These families often face many medical decision points and are supported by intentional and iterative discussions about goals of care. Threats to cohesive goals of care in complex pediatric illness include prognostic uncertainty, diffusion of medical responsibility, individual family context, and blended goals of care. This article offers strategies for addressing each of these challenges—in all cases success involves recognizing how standard care approaches need adaptations to meet the needs of children with serious/complex illness.

CLINICS CARE POINTS

- Creating cohesive goals of care in complex pediatric illness may be threatened by a misaligned understanding of a family's values and desires.
- Mitigating barriers to cohesive goals of care requires attention to team unity around prognosis and outcome(s) and in-depth exploration of family context, in addition to clear and consistent communication.
- Blended goals of care may be a way to meet some expectations, but not all, for families and clinicians alike who may have different viewpoints about the best course of action.

DISCLOSURE

None.

REFERENCES

1. Kuo DZ, Houtrow AJ. Council On Children With D. Recognition and Management of Medical Complexity. Pediatrics 2016;138(6). https://doi.org/10.1542/peds.2016-3021.
2. Cohen E, Kuo DZ, Agrawal R, et al. Children with medical complexity: an emerging population for clinical and research initiatives. Pediatrics 2011;127(3):529–38.
3. Shapiro MC, Henderson CM, Hutton N, et al. Defining Pediatric Chronic Critical Illness for Clinical Care, Research, and Policy. Hosp Pediatr 2017;7(4):236–44.
4. Guttmann K, Kelley A, Weintraub A, et al. Defining Neonatal Serious Illness. J Palliat Med 2022;25(11):1655–60.
5. Rogozinski L, Young A, Grybauskas C, et al. Point Prevalence of Children Hospitalized With Chronic Critical Illness in the General Inpatient Units. Hosp Pediatr 2019;9(7):545–9.
6. Boss RD, Henderson CM, Weiss EM, et al. The Changing Landscape in Pediatric Hospitals: A Multicenter Study of How Pediatric Chronic Critical Illness Impacts NICU Throughput. Am J Perinatol 2020. https://doi.org/10.1055/s-0040-1718572.

7. Shapiro MC, Boss RD, Donohue PK, et al. A snapshot of chronic critical illness in pediatric intensive care units. J Pediatr Intensive Care 2021.

8. Berry JG, Goodman DM, Coller RJ, et al. Association of Home Respiratory Equipment and Supply Use with Health Care Resource Utilization in Children. J Pediatr 2019;207:169–175 e2.

9. Secunda K, Wirpsa MJ, Neely KJ, et al. Use and Meaning of "Goals of Care" in the Healthcare Literature: a Systematic Review and Qualitative Discourse Analysis. J Gen Intern Med 2020;35(5):1559–66.

10. Boss RD, Henderson CM, Raisanen JC, et al. Family Experiences Deciding For and Against Pediatric Home Ventilation. J Pediatr 2021;229:223–31.

11. Aite L, Zaccara A, Trucchi A, et al. When uncertainty generates more anxiety than severity: the prenatal experience with cystic adenomatoid malformation of the lung. J Perinat Med 2009;37(5):539–42.

12. Bogetz JF, Munjapara V, Henderson CM, et al. Home mechanical ventilation for children with severe neurological impairment: Parents' perspectives on clinician counselling. Dev Med Child Neurol 2022. https://doi.org/10.1111/dmcn.15151.

13. Boss RD, Lemmon ME, Arnold RM, et al. Communicating prognosis with parents of critically ill infants: direct observation of clinician behaviors. J Perinatol 2017;37(11):1224–9.

14. Elkinton JR. Medicine and the quality of life. Ann Intern Med 1966;64(3):711–4.

15. Payot A. Best interest standards do not correlate with the reality of physicians' decision making in life and death choices. Evid Based Nurs 2012;15(1):9.

16. Saigal S, Stoskopf BL, Feeny D, et al. Differences in preferences for neonatal outcomes among health care professionals, parents, and adolescents. JAMA 1999;281(21):1991–7.

17. Bogetz JF, Boss RD, Lemmon ME. Communicating With Families of Children With Severe Neurological Impairment. J Pain Symptom Manage 2022;63(2):e264–6.

18. Tate T. Pediatric Suffering and the Burden of Proof. Pediatrics 2020;146(Suppl 1):S70–4.

19. Miller KE, Coleman RD, Eisenberg L, et al. Unilateral Withdrawal of Life-sustaining Therapy in a Severely Impaired Child. Pediatrics 2018;142(5). https://doi.org/10.1542/peds.2018-0131.

20. Boss RD, Hutton N, Griffin PL, et al. Novel legislation for pediatric advance directives: surveys and focus groups capture parent and clinician perspectives. Palliat Med 2015;29(4):346–53.

21. Liberman DB, Pham PK, Nager AL. Pediatric advance directives: parents' knowledge, experience, and preferences. Pediatrics 2014;134(2):e436–43.

22. Wharton RH, Levine KR, Buka S, et al. Advance care planning for children with special health care needs: a survey of parental attitudes. Pediatrics 1996;97(5):682–7.

23. Lotz JD, Daxer M, Jox RJ, et al. "Hope for the best, prepare for the worst": A qualitative interview study on parents' needs and fears in pediatric advance care planning. Palliat Med 2017;31(8):764–71.

24. Fischer P, Krueger JI, Greitemeyer T, et al. The bystander-effect: a meta-analytic review on bystander intervention in dangerous and non-dangerous emergencies. Psychol Bull 2011;137(4):517–37.

25. Stavert RR, Lott JP. The bystander effect in medical care. N Engl J Med 2013;368(1):8–9.

26. Marcus KL, Henderson CM, Boss RD. Chronic Critical Illness in Infants and Children: A Speculative Synthesis on Adapting ICU Care to Meet the Needs of Long-Stay Patients. Pediatr Crit Care Med 2016;17(8):743–52.

27. Kuo DZ, Cohen E, Agrawal R, et al. A national profile of caregiver challenges among more medically complex children with special health care needs. Arch Pediatr Adolesc Med 2011;165(11):1020–6.

28. Kuo DZ, McAllister JW, Rossignol L, et al. Care Coordination for Children With Medical Complexity: Whose Care Is It, Anyway? Pediatrics 2018;141(Suppl 3): S224–32.

29. Cohen E, Berry JG, Sanders L, et al. Status Complexicus? The Emergence of Pediatric Complex Care. Pediatrics 2018;141(Suppl 3):S202–11.

30. Rieger EY, Kushner JNS, Sriram V, et al. Primary care physician involvement during hospitalisation: a qualitative analysis of perspectives from frequently hospitalised patients. BMJ Open 2021;11(12). e053784.

31. Shapiro MC, Donohue PK, Kudchadkar SR, et al. Professional Responsibility, Consensus, and Conflict: A Survey of Physician Decisions for the Chronically Critically Ill in Neonatal and Pediatric Intensive Care Units. Pediatr Crit Care Med 2017;18(9):e415–22.

32. Henderson CM, Wilfond BS, Boss RD. Bringing Social Context Into the Conversation About Pediatric Long-term Ventilation. Hosp Pediatr 2018. https://doi.org/10.1542/hpeds.2016-0168.

33. Stein RE, Siegel MJ, Bauman LJ. Double jeopardy: what social risk adds to biomedical risk in understanding child health and health care utilization. Acad Pediatr 2010;10(3):165–71.

34. Henderson CM, Raisanen JC, Shipman KJ, et al. Life with pediatric home ventilation: Expectations versus experience. Pediatr Pulmonol 2021;56(10):3366–73.

35. Carnevale FA, Alexander E, Davis M, et al. Daily living with distress and enrichment: the moral experience of families with ventilator-assisted children at home. Pediatrics 2006;117(1):e48–60.

36. Ong T, Liu CC, Elder L, et al. The Trach Safe Initiative: A Quality Improvement Initiative to Reduce Mortality among Pediatric Tracheostomy Patients. Otolaryngol Head Neck Surg 2020;163(2):221–31.

37. Edwards JD, Kun SS, Keens TG. Outcomes and causes of death in children on home mechanical ventilation via tracheostomy: an institutional and literature review. J Pediatr 2010;157(6):955–959 e2.

38. Brehaut JC, Garner RE, Miller AR, et al. Changes over time in the health of caregivers of children with health problems: growth-curve findings from a 10-year Canadian population-based study. Am J Public Health 2011;101(12):2308–16.

39. Wright-Sexton LA, Compretta CE, Blackshear C, et al. Isolation in Parents and Providers of Children With Chronic Critical Illness. Pediatr Crit Care Med 2020; 21(8):e530–7.

40. Hebert LM, Watson AC, Madrigal V, et al. Discussing Benefits and Risks of Tracheostomy: What Physicians Actually Say. Pediatr Crit Care Med 2017;18(12): e592–7.

41. Available at: www.Family-Reflections.com. Accessed April 7, 2023.

42. Available at: www.CourageousParentsNetwork.com. Accessed April 7, 2023.

43. Caruso Brown AE, Ciurria J. "Prix Fixe" or "A La Carte"? Pediatric Decision Making When the Goals of Care Lie in the Zone of Parental Discretion. J Clin Ethics 2021; 32(4):299–306.

44. McDougall R, Gillam L, Spriggs M, et al. The zone of parental discretion and the complexity of paediatrics: A response to Alderson. Clin Ethics 2018;13(4):172–4.

45. Ullrich C, Morrison RS. Pediatric palliative care research comes of age: what we stand to learn from children with life-threatening illness. J Palliat Med 2013;16(4): 334–6.

46. McGraw SA, Truog RD, Solomon MZ, et al. "I was able to still be her mom"–parenting at end of life in the pediatric intensive care unit. Pediatr Crit Care Med 2012;13(6):e350–6.

47. Lindley LC, Cozad MJ, Mack JW, et al. Effectiveness of Pediatric Concurrent Hospice Care to Improve Continuity of Care. Am J Hosp Palliat Care 2022;39(10):1129–36.

48. Lipstein EA, Brinkman WB, Britto MT. What is known about parents' treatment decisions? A narrative review of pediatric decision making. Med Decis Making 2012;32(2):246–58.

Consent and Assent in Pediatric Research

D. Micah Hester, PhD*, Skye A. Miner, PhD

KEYWORDS

- Pediatric research • Assent • Therapeutic misconception • Common rule

KEY POINTS

- Pediatric populations often cannot consent to their own research participation; thus, parental permission is often required.
- The Common Rule, Subpart D outlines special protections for including pediatric populations in research.
- Although assent from the potential pediatric population is not always required by the regulations, it is an important ethical consideration in including pediatric populations in research.
- Creating a process of assent in pediatric research respects children's developing autonomy and helps them articulate their values.

CASE

Sonya is a 15-year-old girl who was diagnosed with acute myeloid leukemia (AML) when she was 11 years. In the last 2 years, her parents have been diligent with her care, getting her to appointments, keeping her routine with medications. But unfortunately, two rounds of chemotherapy have failed. She received a bone marrow transplant 18 months ago, but she has been brought to the hospital because of fatigue and general flu-like symptoms that have lasted more than a week.

Sonya's oncologist suspects that this is another relapse into AML and having few clinical options tells Sonya's parents that there is a clinical trial testing the latest therapies at another center about 5 to 6 hours away by car that Sonya should be eligible to participate in and that it is as good a chance as they have at a cure for Sonya.

However, when this is explained to Sonya, she states, "I am too tired, everything makes me sick, and I know I'm dying anyway; so, I just want to stay at home."

INTRODUCTION

The case raises several ethical questions surrounding the inclusion of pediatric participants in therapeutic research trials, including the possibility that Sonya's physician is

Department of Medical Humanities and Bioethics, College of Medicine, University of Arkansas for Medical Science, 4301 West Markham Street, #646, Little Rock, AR 72205, USA
* Corresponding author.
E-mail address: dmhester@uams.edu

Pediatr Clin N Am 71 (2024) 83–92
https://doi.org/10.1016/j.pcl.2023.08.003
0031-3955/24/© 2023 Elsevier Inc. All rights reserved.

approaching the clinical trial as if it is clinical therapy; the concern that Sonya's parents do not fully understand that they are being asked to allow Sonya to be part of a research trial aiming at generalizable knowledge; and the ability of Sonya herself to assent to research.

We will use Sonya's case to explore the ethics of clinical research with children and adolescents. Although research with pediatric populations has special considerations to ensure the protection of certain vulnerabilities, pediatric research is still necessary to advance our understanding of a condition/disease that only impacts children,[1,2] a condition/disease that impacts children and adults differently,[2] a drug/intervention that may have different effects on pediatric populations,[3] a psychological/sociologic phenomenon that is relevant to children,[4] and pediatric affects that may inform treatment of an adult-onset condition.[2,4] Troubling, though, in the case of pediatric populations, roughly 60% of new pediatric-relevant medications lack pediatric prescribing information 5 years after Federal Drug Administration (FDA) approval.[5] This lack of testing puts children at even greater risk than adults when they receive clinical care. As such, it is important to create scientifically valid and ethically supportable research that includes children as participants. However, pediatric research does pose particular ethical challenges.

In this article, we first explain the differences between clinical care and research investigations, paying special attention to how therapeutic misconception and therapeutic optimism may present differently when parents are asked to provide permission for the child's involvement in research. Then, the regulatory environment that governs research with children will be discussed. In this discussion, we review requirement of parental permission and when waivers of parental permission by the institutional reveiw board (IRB) may be appropriate. Next, we review the concept of assent and dissent in research, documenting the procedural requirement and recommending a process to address this requirement. Finally, special circumstances will be discussed.

In our case, Sonya's physician, her parents, and possibly Sonya herself may be conflating important differences between research and clinical care. Like many patients, Sonya is eligible to be enrolled in a clinical trial because of her specific diagnosis; however, the considerations and concerns that the clinician, researcher, Sonya, and her parents must have in deciding whether or not Sonya should participate in the trial are different than the considerations and concerns for deciding whether to provide medicines or other interventions in clinical care.

The first consideration regards the status of potential benefit for Sonya. Unlike in clinical care where the physician is tasked with focusing on providing individualized, beneficial information and interventions for the specific patient in front of them, researchers are tasked with ensuring that the patient understands the purpose of research—namely to develop "generalizable knowledge" rather than benefitting any particular patient. In generating "generalizable knowledge," the potential benefit to any individual participant in research is unknown and the investigator must follow a carefully defined protocol that places the participant in the role of a data point. As such, research, as compared with clinical care, focuses less on individual well-being and runs a significant risk of dehumanizing the participant as primarily a vector for information and insight.

Sonya and Sonya's parents, thus, like any other research participant, must be carefully and fully informed that Sonya would be shifting her role from patient to participant, which entails potential for a lack of individual benefit to Sonya. Without this recognition, Sonya and her parents are at risk for the therapeutic misconception in that they may not fully understand "that the defining purpose of clinical research is to produce generalizable knowledge, regardless of whether [Sonya] may potentially benefit from the intervention under study or from aspects of the clinical trial."[6] Therapeutic misconception, thus, violates the ethical norm of "respect for persons" where in order to be properly informed about one's research participation (or to give permission for a child to participate), one must fully understand the risks and benefits of participating.

Establishing an informed consent process that ensures that potential participants understand that they are participating in research so that they do not overestimate the benefit that they could receive through their participation has been called for by multiple research ethics statements. However, such statements tend to be adult-focused, with documents like the Nuremberg Code[7] specifically stating that only the participant him/herself can give consent. As children are not typically treated (in the United States, at least) as having the authority to consent for themselves, pediatric research seems untenable under these early documents. Subsequent documents, such as the Declaration of Helsinki[8] (1964; current rev 2013), established the authority of a legally authorized representative (such as parents of minors) to give consent for research.

Despite the ability for Sonya's parents to provide consent for her participation, there are questions about the limits, exceptions, or conditions placed on that decisional authority, especially when the child, such as Sonya, raises objections about their participation. Of course, in clinical care, a child's objection may not bar treatment considered to be beneficial. However, because many trials are not designed to benefit the individual child, the individual child's dissent to participate in research should be given different ethical consideration than in clinical care. The regulatory limitations with regard to the types of trials that minors participate in are guardrails that delineate how to engage children about their participation and also ensure that children's inability to provide fully informed consent does not unduly increase their vulnerability.

Vulnerability of Minors and the Regulatory Environment

The necessity of informed consent is not only laid out in the Nuremberg Code and the Declaration of Helsinki, but it also documented in "The Belmont Report"[9] (here on out, Belmont) as a research application (ie, practice) that is tied to the research principle or "prescriptive judgments" of Respect for Persons. Specifically, the report states, "Respect for persons requires that subjects, to the degree that they are *capable*, be given the opportunity to choose what shall or shall not happen to them. This opportunity is provided when adequate standards for informed consent are satisfied."[9]

Of course, the caveat in the provision matters—namely, the "capability" of "subjects" does vary by degrees. For this reason, they note later:

Special provision may need to be made when comprehension is severely limited—for example, by conditions of immaturity or mental disability. Each class of subjects that one might consider as incompetent (eg, infants and young children, mentally disabled patients, the terminally ill, and the comatose) should be considered on its own terms.[9]

Belmont, then recognizes that "children" (we shall use the term "minors," as well) comprise a "class of subjects" for which "special provisions" may be needed when determining research participation.

To understand the cultural presumption in the United States on a minor consenting for themselves, one must take into consideration the fact that human beings are a species with a long developmental period from infancy to adulthood. For the first 2 decades of life (at least), humans go through significant, even fundamental, changes physiologically, psychologically, and socially. During this development period, human cognition is peculiarly vulnerable—as the ability to reason through difficult circumstances is often undermined by underdeveloped logical skills, lack of experience, lack of foresight, and waves of emotion. These underdeveloped skills are problematic to achieving consent because it is the ability to reason through, understand, and appreciate the gravity of the considerations that make up decisional capacity. Because minors are seen to lack capacity to make complex decisions and be held fully accountable for their decisions and actions, most state laws do not allow persons less than the age of 18 years to have the authority to make decisions for themselves. The lack of legal authority predicated on developmental vulnerability, then, has implications for participation of minors in research and the regulations that govern research.

Currently regulated by the Common Rule (45 CFR 46),[10] Subpart D of these regulations speaks to research with/about children. The Common Rule tasks IRBs to determine the risks that the children will face regarding their participation, categorize that risk, and then set up adequate procedures for informed consent by parents and assent (to the extent possible) by children themselves. The Common Rule categorizes pediatric risk into three risk categories (1) not involving greater than minimal risk (section 404); (2) involving greater than minimal risk but presenting the prospect of direct benefit to the individual subjects (section 405); and (3) involving greater than minimal risk and no prospect of direct benefit to individual subjects, but likely to yield generalizable knowledge about the subject's disorder or condition (section 406). Importantly, these risk categories demand an assessment of risk with the weighing of the potential benefit, either to the child or others like them. In establishing the importance of generalizable knowledge, the Common Rule also provides permission for research that is not otherwise approvable but presents an opportunity to understand, prevent, or alleviate a serious problem affecting the health or welfare of children (section 407).

Section 408 of the Common Rule (Subpart D) goes on to provide the process of informed consent should be achieved with parents. The expectation is "that adequate provisions are made for soliciting the permission of each child's parents or guardian" (mirroring subpart A's requirement of informed consent for adults). The number of parents who must provide permission depends on the level of risk of the study (46.406 and 46.407 require two-parent permission) and the reasonability of obtaining the permission from both parents.

These regulatory provisions are attempts to mitigate the vulnerability of the minor participant, particularly when the risks are identifiable and significant, but the research lacks prospective benefits to participants. However, the primary protection comes from parents themselves exercising their moral responsibilities to agree only to research that meets with their child's interests.

Parental Authority and Permission

Although the Common Rule reflects other laws that provide for parental authority in decision-making over their children, this authority also creates certain ethical expectations for parents. In particular, parents are expected to provide for their children's basic needs (shelter, food, education, and so forth), striving for doing best by their children, in light of the social and environmental conditions in which the family operates. Certainly, one basic need for minors is their health, and when a child is ill or injured, parents are expected to do what will make their child better, when that is possible.

With no detailed history of Sonya and her family, let us assume that Sonya's parents have taken their parental responsibilities and authority seriously, attending to Sonya's basic needs and caring for her during all stages of her illness. Now, however, they encounter the decision to enroll their daughter in a clinical research trial. Although this decision is a new inflection point for parental consideration, in fact, this decision is not remarkable from the standpoint of pediatric oncology; approximately 50% of pediatric oncology patients less than 15 years old are in a clinical research trial.[11] Although such trials are often labeled "therapeutic," as noted above, research differs fundamentally from clinical care itself—namely, clinical care aims at the well-being of the individual patient, whereas research aims at generalizable knowledge. As such, then, research protocols challenge the determination about what is "best" for the child themselves, given that research is never directly about the well-being of any particular participant.

Now, in adult-based determinations for research participation, it is recognized that the adult with reasonable decisional capacity should be allowed to exercise their autonomy by agreeing to be part of research, even if it will be of no benefit (even create risk) for them. However, as described above, lacking capacity, *children cannot make this decision for themselves directly*. Parents, then, provide the permission (aka, "parental consent") for their child participate in a research protocol, and yet, doing so puts parents in a tenuous moral position regarding their duty to protect their children from harm and aim at doing best for their child.

To make a decision about their child's participation, parents must receive all information about a clinical trial, including the possibility that their child may not benefit from their participation, may have heightened risks, and may even be harmed as a participant. The provision of permission for a child to engage in risky research, thus, may seem to violate a central ethical tenent of ethical parental decision-making where a narrow view of parental authority may require *only* actions that meet recognizable "best interests" of the child, avoiding foreseeable undue harm. This risk-avoidance strategy, however, ignores the potential benefits of research participation to the child to others and to science. Although parents may weigh the benefits of their child's participation differently, their decision to permit their child to participate should include a consideration of their child's current (and possibly future) values and may include as a factor what kinds of values they wish to instill in their child (eg, altruism).

Minor Assent and Dissent

Although parental permission is guided by ethical norms and regulatory language, the individual participating in research is the minor themselves. That is, the child will be the one undergoing any investigation or intervention on behalf of the research protocol, not the parent(s). In light of this, Belmont notes, "Even for these persons, however, respect requires giving them the opportunity to choose to the extent they are able, whether or not to participate in research. The objections of these subjects to involvement should be honored, unless the research entails providing them a therapy unavailable elsewhere."

What follows from these insights is that *participants in research should be allowed to participate* in research (from the recruitment and consent process until the close of the protocol) to the degree possible given their cognitive, psychological, and physiologic conditions. The participation of minors in the informed consent process minimally requires them to understand the research question. This understanding, however, is often limited to the child's current intellectual and developmental abilities.[12] Thus, to assess an individual child's understanding of the research material, one should also ensure that the material and discussions are developmentally appropriate.[13]

Although some may suggest that material should be presented in an age-appropriate way, the focus on age rather than development ignores the individuality of childhood development in that certain circumstances may make a child more prone to understanding complex medical information, even at a young age.[14] For example, imagine Sonya was first diagnosed with AML at age 6 years was treated for a period of time and went into remission until the age of 8 years. Her understanding of her disease and even the medications to treat the disease would be different from an 8-year-old who has rarely encountered the medical system.

The individuality and contextual factors that impact the ability of a child to understand the research may be one reason why there is a lack of consensus on the age at which children can appropriately understand consent. However, some research suggests that all children without development delay should be asked for their assent above the age of 12 years and children between the ages of 10 and 12 years should be assessed individually.[15] There are several tools that have been developed to help researchers establish the assent process, including comic books,[16] educational videos,[17] and other multimedia approaches.[18] These tools have been used to provide developmentally appropriate information and have often been shown to improve the understanding of the study procedures as compared with a traditional IRB-approved form.[19]

Although there are different modes of engaging minors in the assent process, how researchers should incorporate this engagement as assent or dissent is debated. Diekema[20] argues that "assent should not be equated with consent" in that "the purpose of assent is not to treat children as if they are capable of making decisions that are as fully informed and autonomous as those made by adults." That is, assent and the assenting process provides benefits to children, including helping develop their autonomy and feeling like they are "heard" as part of the research process.[20] The process of assent then allows children to express their viewpoints and for these objections or permissions to be taken into consideration.[21]

This, too, is recognized in The Common Rule under the concept of "assent." According to The Common Rule, "Assent means a child's affirmative agreement to participate in research" (sec 402). We will refer to this as the "product" definition of "assent," wherein assent means a (final) determination by a child agreeing to be part of research. Further, though, the regulations indicate that "adequate provisions [should be] made for soliciting the assent of the children, when…children are capable of providing assent" (sec 408). We shall call this the "process" requirement for "assent" as this statement requires that investigators create conditions and processes for determining what the child themselves wants with regard to research participation. Although both explications of "assent" are important in different contexts, these two versions of "assent" in the regulations create an ambiguity in the protections' provisions under sections 404 to 407.

Although sections 404 to 407 all require that "adequate provisions are made for soliciting the assent of the children" (process), the ambiguity becomes apparent especially under section 405 research. Under section 408 regarding "assent," the regulations state that when "the intervention or procedure involved in the research holds out a prospect of direct benefit [research under section 405] that is important to the health or well-being of the children and is available only in the context of the research, the assent of the children is not a necessary condition for proceeding with the research."

Thus, it would seem that the regulations under section 405 both allow research to proceed without minor "assent" and yet require soliciting "assent." This only makes sense, however, if we accept one of two interpretations of the regulations.

1. When assent is set aside for section 405 research, this also sets aside the requirement for "soliciting assent." This position makes sense because there would seem to be no reason to solicit something that has no weight in the outcome of the decision to participate. However, two things speak against this reading.
   a. The regulations explicitly state under section 405 that provisions for assent should be made.
   b. It may be misleading to say that the "solicitation" is valueless even when there is no final "affirmation" to be captured.

2. The regulations purposefully require assent *processes* even when the *product* may not be the final determination of whether a child participates in research. This position makes sense given the analysis of two different versions of assent in the regulations. This analytical bifurcation, then, places emphasis on *the importance of assent processes which, as we noted earlier, treat the minor as a participant in research* to the extent they are capable, whereas they recognize that some situations posed by research fall within the purview of parental authority given the complex considerations that a child may not be able to adjudicate adequately for themselves.

Treating the minor as a participant in research, to the extent they are capable, helps to respect the minor's developing capacity and autonomy. In studies of minors who were included in research, most appreciate the inclusion and make decisions that are in conversation with their parents.[13,22] Thus, although we have presented a case where the minor herself and the parents are seemingly in disagreement about Sonya's enrollment, the pressure to participate because of parents' influence may only occur a small minority of the time—for example, 15% of the minors in Grady and colleagues's[13] study on assent felt like their parents gave them "no voice regarding their participation." Although differences in opinions about enrollment in a potentially beneficial trial may only occur a minority of the time and regulations do not require a child's permission, ethically their dissent should be strongly considered as they will be the participants and by including their "voice" in research may be an important in helping the child develop into an autonomous adult. Thus, the first step in resolving the case between Sonya and her parents is allowing Sonya to speak freely with her parents about her concerns regarding participation in research and for her parents to provide reasons for wanting her to participate. In listening to her concerns, her parents may adjust their perspective surrounding her participation. Alternatively, Sonya's parents may suggest values and interests or provide an alternative perspective about Sonya's participation that may make Sonya reconsider her own participation. These conversations may resolve the tension between parent and child and also serve to respect the child's developing autonomy.

SPECIAL CIRCUMSTANCES REGARDING CONSENT AND ASSENT

Despite the ethical importance of the inclusion of children in the consent process, IRBs and researchers have discretion in the requirements for researchers to obtain assent from the adolescent and parental permission from the parents. As noted above, research that involves the prospect of direct benefit (section 405), a child's dissent may be overridden by parents if the IRB determines the therapeutic trial offers the a possible benefit to the participant not otherwise available outside the trial. However, what is considered prospective, direct benefit can depend on the IRB that reviews the study.[23] In addition, IRBs have discretion in requiring parental permission if the "study is designed for conditions or for a subject population for which parental or guardian permission is not a reasonable requirement to protect the subjects (for example, neglected or abused children)" (45 CFR 46.408). This waiver for parental permission may also be granted if the study involves circumstances, which are clearly outside of parental control. These waivers are intended to protect existing vulnerabilities in children (eg, privacy) and allow them to make decisions aligned with the child's current decision-making responsibilities. Although these waivers provide for exceptions to the current federal regulations, they also mean that IRBs have discretion to determine the necessity of both parental permission and child assent.

The variability of IRB determinations is further complicated by state laws which may allow minors to consent for themselves. For example, in California, minors older than the age of 12 are able to consent to medical treatment that involves drug-misuse, sexual assault, sexually transmitted disease, and outpatient mental health services.[24] Thus, research that involves the testing of certain interventions related to these areas may also be considered research in which the minor (who has capacity) can consent for themselves. The ability for a minor to determine their participation in research involving these behaviors or decisions respects the minor's privacy and may also be captured under a waiver of parental permission as outlined by 45 CFR 46.408.

In thinking about these exceptions, it is important to note that they are rooted in many of the same ethical principles that require parental permission and childhood assent, namely they arise for the importance of *protecting* children involved in research. As such, exceptions provided by the IRB and the state law are aimed at ensuring that the child's participation in research does not reveal information to the parent that may be intentionally kept private. Again, childhood assent is rooted in the idea that assent allows for children to develop their autonomy and be participants to the extent possible in the research process. Thus, in areas of life where children may have already developed the capacity to make decisions, it is reasonable to allow them to make their own research decisions as well.

SUMMARY

The process of soliciting a minor's assent has moral import, even if it is not always required by the current regulations. Ethically, the process provides for the child's opinion to be heard, for respecting their developing capacity and involving the child as a participant in research. Of course, the extent to which a child should be involved in the assent process depends on the age, experience, and maturity of the child. This put the onus on researchers to enable a minor's understanding of a research protocol by providing the trial information in a developmentally appropriate way. Although a minor's assent is an important process, their dissent may not be determinative. Instead, researchers and parents should engage in a discussion about the dissent. During this conversation, it is important to ensure that the child and the parents understand the risks and benefits of participation and do not conflate the research process with clinical care (ie, cause therapeutic misconception).

Returning, then, to our case, the researcher should first facilitate a conversation with Sonya and her parents. Her parents may be misunderstanding the purpose of research, conflating Sonya's participation with another clinical option. This therapeutic misconception should first be resolved by providing the appropriate risk and benefit information to Sonya and her family and by explaining the purpose of the trial, namely that it is to generate generalizable knowledge. After this conversation, the researcher should solicit both Sonya and her parents' understanding and perspective. During this conversation, it will be important to highlight shared values and perspectives as well as understand the nature of any remaining disagreement. The purpose of this conversation is to ensure both that the parents and Sonya understand the research and that Sonya herself feels heard. However, despite the ethical need for this conversation, the case describes a research trial that likely has atrue prospect of direct benefit for Sonya. Thus, Sonya's affirmative agreement to participate in the trial would likely not be required by the IRB, leaving final decision-making authority to her parents.

Research with pediatric populations carries certain ethical considerations. Regulations, including The Common Rule, attempt to put procedures in place to ensure that ethical processes are followed and that the vulnerabilities of children are protected.

These include requirements for including pediatric populations in all phases of research, including the consent/assent process. The ethical importance of inclusion of pediatric populations in both research and the assent/consent process ensures that despite children's vulnerabilities, they are recognized as human participants with developing autonomy and values. Thus, it is important for researchers, clinicians, and IRBs to recognize both the vulnerabilities of this special population and the ways that inclusion of pediatric populations can advance scientific discovery.

CLINICS CARE POINTS

- Know the regulations: Parents have wide authority to determine medical care for their minor children; however, research ethics and regulations place limits on parental authority.
- Respect and Assent: Minors, to the extent they are psychologically and intellectually capable, should be included in decisions to enroll in research trials.
- Wide Discretion: IRBs may insist on additional protections for minors, depending on concerns for a participant's safety or, even, adherence to the protocol.

DISCLOSURE

DMH is a member of the National Cancer Institute's Pediatric Central Institutional Review Board.

REFERENCES

1. Klassen TP, Hartling L, Hamm M, et al. StaR Child Health: an initiative for RCTs in children. Lancet 2009;374(9698):1310–2.
2. Speer EM, Lee LK, Bourgeois FT, et al. The state and future of pediatric research—an introductory overview. Pediatr Res 2023. https://doi.org/10.1038/s41390-022-02439-4.
3. Joseph PD, Craig JC, Caldwell PH. Clinical trials in children. Br J Clin Pharmacol 2015;79(3):357–69.
4. National Institutes of Health. Inclusion Across the Lifespan, 2023. https://grants.nih.gov/policy/inclusion/lifespan.htm. Accessed March 30, 2023.
5. Carmack M, Hwang T, Bourgeois FT. Pediatric Drug Policies Supporting Safe And Effective Use Of Therapeutics In Children: A Systematic Analysis. Health Aff 2020;39(10):1799–805. https://doi.org/10.1377/hlthaff.2020.00198.
6. Henderson GE, Churchill LR, Davis AM, et al. Clinical trials and medical care: defining the therapeutic misconception. PLoS Med 2007;4(11):e324. https://doi.org/10.1371/journal.pmed.0040324.
7. Nuremberg Code. 1947. Available at: https://ori.hhs.gov/content/chapter-3-The-Protection-of-Human-Subjects-nuremberg-code-directives-human-experimentation. Accessed August 31, 2023.
8. World Medical Association. Declaration of Helsinki. 2013 (1964).
9. National Commission for the Protection of Human Subjects. The Belmont report: ethical principles and guidelines for the protection of human subjects of research. Vol. 1. 1978.
10. The Common Rule 45 CFR 46. 2018 (1981).
11. Schapira MM, Stevens EM, Sharpe JE, et al. Outcomes among pediatric patients with cancer who are treated on trial versus off trial: A matched cohort study. Cancer 2020;126(15):3471–82.

12. Wendler DS. Assent in paediatric research: theoretical and practical considerations. J Med Ethics 2006;32(4):229–34.
13. Grady C, Wiener L, Abdoler E, et al. Assent in research: the voices of adolescents. J Adolesc Health 2014;54(5):515–20. https://doi.org/10.1016/j.jadohealth.2014.02.005.
14. Scherer DG, Brody JL, Annett RD, et al. Empirically Derived Knowledge on Adolescent Assent to Pediatric Biomedical Research. AJOB Primary Research 2013;4(3):15–26. https://doi.org/10.1080/21507716.2013.806967.
15. Hein IM, De Vries MC, Troost PW, et al. Informed consent instead of assent is appropriate in children from the age of twelve: Policy implications of new findings on children's competence to consent to clinical research. BMC Med Ethics 2015; 16(1):76. https://doi.org/10.1186/s12910-015-0067-z.
16. Massetti T, Crocetta TB, Guarnieri R, et al. A didactic approach to presenting verbal and visual information to children participating in research protocols: the comic book informed assent. Clinics 2018;73:e207.
17. Nuffield Council on Bioethics. Health research: making the right decision for me, 2023. https://www.youtube.com/watch?v=6yaKwLG_vlE. Accessed March 30, 2023.
18. O'Lonergan TA, Forster-Harwood JE. Novel approach to parental permission and child assent for research: improving comprehension. Pediatrics 2011;127(5): 917–24.
19. Weisleder P. Helping Them Decide: A Scoping Review of Interventions Used to Help Minors Understand the Concept and Process of Assent. Mini Review. Frontiers in Pediatrics 2020;February(07):8.
20. Diekema DS. Taking Children Seriously: What's so Important about Assent? Am J Bioeth 2003;3(4):25–6.
21. Giesbertz NAA, Bredenoord AL, van Delden JJM. Clarifying assent in pediatric research. Eur J Hum Genet 2014;22(2):266–9.
22. Pervola J, Myers MF, McGowan ML, et al. Giving adolescents a voice: the types of genetic information adolescents choose to learn and why. Genet Med 2019; 21(4):965–71. https://doi.org/10.1038/s41436-018-0320-1.
23. Shah S, Whittle A, Wilfond B, et al. How do institutional review boards apply the federal risk and benefit standards for pediatric research? JAMA 2004;291(4): 476–82. https://doi.org/10.1001/jama.291.4.476.
24. California Legislation. California Family Code. 1994.

Management of Uncertainty in Everyday Pediatric Care

Nicholas A. Jabre, MD, MS[a],*, Margaret R. Moon, MD, MPH[b]

KEYWORDS

- Uncertainty in pediatrics • Shared decision-making • Managing uncertainty
- Tolerating uncertainty • Child's best interest

KEY POINTS

- Uncertainty in health care may be due to limitations in personal knowledge, existing knowledge, and difficulty distinguishing between the two.
- Types of uncertainty that have been described include scientific, practical, and personal uncertainty, and each may develop from issues of probability, ambiguity, and complexity.
- Pediatricians encounter additional uncertainty related to the limited decision-making capacity of children and to the integral role of families in pediatric care.
- Clinicians may approach uncertainty in different ways: some with a higher tolerance and some with a lower tolerance for its presence.
- Effective management of uncertainty involves: (1) acknowledging its presence, (2) minimizing uncertainty when possible—while still accepting that some uncertainty must be tolerated, and (3) recognizing the interpersonal nature of uncertainty and the role of pediatricians to navigate it together with families.

CASE 1

A pediatrician at a busy suburban practice is seeing a 4-year-old boy and his mother to establish care. During the visit, the mother states that her son has had a recurrent cough since starting daycare 3 months ago. She states that his cough is exacerbated by viral illnesses, which he seems to acquire every 2 to 3 weeks, and that his symptoms are sometimes accompanied by wheezing and significant respiratory distress. The young boy has been taken to urgent care and the local emergency room (ER) on numerous occasions, where he typically received treatment with azithromycin, amoxicillin, and albuterol. However, none of these medications have led to any significant perceived benefit. During his most recent visit to the emergency room last week, the ER physician told the mother that "her son might have asthma" and started the

[a] Division of Pediatric Pulmonology, Johns Hopkins All Children's Hospital, 601 5th Street South, Suite C780, St Petersburg, FL 33701, USA; [b] Johns Hopkins Berman Institute of Bioethics, 1809 Ashland Avenue, Baltimore, MD 21205, USA
* Corresponding author.
E-mail address: njabre1@jhmi.edu

Pediatr Clin N Am 71 (2024) 93–100
https://doi.org/10.1016/j.pcl.2023.08.004
0031-3955/24/© 2023 Elsevier Inc. All rights reserved.

boy on a course of oral steroids. His mother is understandably concerned about the possibility of this diagnosis, and asks what can be done to stop her child from becoming ill again. She also explained that she could not afford to miss any more days of work, having to take care of her son when he is sent home from daycare due to his cough.

CASE 2

A 6-month-old infant with extreme prematurity was transferred to the neonatal intensive care unit (NICU) of a large children's hospital for continued management of respiratory failure and feeding difficulties. She developed an intraventricular hemorrhage, which was initially identified on head ultrasound at 1 week of age, and her severe dysphagia necessitated placement of a gastrostomy tube. Since birth, she has required gradual escalation of respiratory support, culminating in intubation and mechanical ventilation. Imaging of her lungs showed thick scar formation consistent with severe bronchopulmonary dysplasia. She has failed to wean from the ventilator on several occasions and placement of a tracheostomy tube is now being offered as a treatment option. The infant's family consists of her mother, father, and 9-year-old sibling. Both parents are employed but are currently taking time off from work. They live in a rural part of the state and are currently staying at a local hotel. The infant's mother continually states that she "just wants to get our baby home."

INTRODUCTION/BACKGROUND

Uncertainty permeates all aspects of medicine. It is experienced by all clinicians at various times throughout their careers and poses unique challenges to communicating with families and making decisions.[1] These challenges may include difficulty discerning the trustworthiness of clinical data, knowing whether patients can comprehend ambiguous clinical situations, and recognizing the point at which overthinking becomes counterproductive. Pediatricians face additional challenges related to the values and preferences of families and the impact of treatment decisions on children who have limited capacity to decide what will happen to them.

What is uncertainty in the health-care setting? The concept of uncertainty has been described as the subjective awareness of one's own lack of knowledge[2] and may develop due to limitations in personal knowledge and/or limitations in the field of medicine as a whole.[3] Many types of uncertainty have been described[2] and include uncertainty related to specific diagnoses or disease states, practical issues related to accessing health care, and personal issues dealing with the influence of disease on identity and quality of life.

Pediatricians and other clinicians may approach these uncertainties in a variety of ways. Some may disregard them, choosing to maintain their professional authority over patients. Some may embrace them, seeking to discuss uncertainty with families to better assess their values and treatment goals. The American Academy of Pediatrics (AAP) urges pediatricians to consider the preferences of families, children, and young adults when making medical decisions.[4] Thus, it is essential to acknowledge and discuss sources of uncertainty with children, young adults, and their families to encourage them to participate in the process of shared decision-making.

In this article, we summarize the types of uncertainty in medicine, emphasizing how these may be encountered in pediatric practice. We also describe different ways that pediatricians and other clinicians may approach uncertainty. Finally, we outline a strategy to effectively manage uncertainty in the clinical setting, leveraging it for the benefit of our patients, and learning to take the middle ground between too much and too little tolerance of uncertainty when making decisions together with our patients and their families.

DISCUSSION
Types of Uncertainty

In her seminal study, describing the experience of uncertainty in medical students as they complete their training, sociologist Renee Fox described three types of uncertainty that can be experienced by clinicians.[3] The first type is characterized by incomplete mastery of available information. No clinician can fully comprehend the vastness of medicine, and at some point, each clinician will encounter the limits of his or her own knowledge and experience. Uncertainty in these clinical scenarios can be addressed by consulting colleagues, and/or by searching the literature for existing guidelines and empirical research. The second type of uncertainty relates to limitations in the current state of medical knowledge. Clinicians will inevitably encounter questions that are unanswered, due to insufficient advances in the field. These uncertainties can only be reduced or eliminated by further advances in knowledge; until this happens, this type of uncertainty must be tolerated. The third type of uncertainty relates to the first two and is characterized by the inability to distinguish between them.

The experience of uncertainty in health care is not limited to clinicians, and thus, it is helpful to consider broader taxonomies that categorize the sources of uncertainty and their related issues that can be experienced by clinicians, patients, and families alike. Han and colleagues (2011) characterized uncertainty as being scientific, practical, or personal in nature.[2] Scientific uncertainty deals with unknowns about a given disease-state, including questions about its diagnosis, prognosis, cause, or available treatment options. Practical uncertainty is described as systems-based and involves questions about the competence of one's physician, the quality of a certain health-care institution, or the steps necessary to obtain care. Personal uncertainty is described as patient-focused, and it pertains to the influence of disease on one's well-being, personal identity, and overall outlook on life. Each of the 3 kinds of uncertainty can develop from various sources, including the probability or risk of a given outcome, the ambiguity of available information, and the complexity of the situation at hand.

Pediatricians encounter additional uncertainties related to the limited decision-making capacity of children and the integral role of families in pediatric care. Pediatricians must help families make decisions for their child despite having limited ability to know the child's values and treatment goals. Furthermore, parents may have an incomplete understanding of the implications of treatment decisions on the child and caregivers at home. For example, pediatricians and families may struggle to know how a severe neurologic illness will affect the child's quality of life, their future developmental potential, and the strength of family relationships. For critically ill children who will require technology support, pediatricians and families may even question whether further life-sustaining interventions for the child should be provided. When these uncertainties develop, pediatricians must work together closely with families to determine the child's best interest despite numerous unknowns.

Approaches to Uncertainty

Pediatricians and other clinicians may approach uncertainty in different ways, with approaches depending on their individual comfort with uncertainty and their ability to tolerate its presence.[5] Clinicians who are less tolerant of uncertainty experience anxiety and discomfort with the unknown. These individuals are less honest with their patients and may withhold information from them, which they deem to be too upsetting or confusing. These individuals may also feel compelled to oversimplify information to make it easier to understand and may minimize communication with patients until the situation becomes clearer. In contrast, clinicians who are more tolerant of uncertainty are less bothered by the unknown. Such individuals are more honest with families about the limits of their knowledge. They avoid forcing ambiguous data into predefined narratives or illness-scripts and communicate openly with families to solicit their input and to build trust.

In a classic example of the varying abilities to tolerate uncertainty, medical ethicist Jay Katz describes his conversations with a physician colleague who is less comfortable with uncertainty.[1] The colleague indicated that much remains to be learned about the available treatment options for his patients, and accordingly he allows less scope for dialog about the various choices. He states that "theoretic" conversation has no application in clinical practice. Furthermore, he believes that patients "do not have the capacity to understand such complex matters," and having conversations involving uncertainties "would cause them anxiety and pain." In contrast, Katz imagines approaching the situation much differently by carefully laying out the treatment options, discussing each in detail, and soliciting the patient's preference and reason for their choice. Only then would he offer a treatment recommendation. Katz rationalizes that this approach would prevent patients from feeling pressured by professional authority and would allow the clinician to better explore patients' wishes and expectations.

It seems that intolerance of uncertainty should be avoided. However, neither too little tolerance of uncertainty nor too much tolerance of uncertainty is the more desirable, and each approach has its perils.[5] Clinicians who are too intolerant of uncertainty preclude the possibility of shared decision-making with patients, by avoiding opportunities to incorporate their preferences into the treatment plan. They may also fail to act in a timely fashion due to the overanalysis of ambiguous or incomplete information, thus diminishing their effectiveness as healers. In contrast, clinicians who are too tolerant of uncertainty may discuss too many unknowns with patients and/or reveal too many of their own personal uncertainties, thus diminishing patients' confidence in them.[6] They may also risk becoming complacent, and they may not be motivated to consult colleagues and/or research answers to improve their knowledge. Furthermore, they may act prematurely either when the degree of uncertainty is too great or when more time and clarity are actually needed. Thus, there is likely an ideal middle ground, between low and high tolerance of uncertainty, for any given situation that maintains patients' confidence in providers while maximizing collaboration and trust.

Pediatricians may struggle to find balance between these two approaches—of reticence or disclosure. They may feel compelled to communicate in unambiguous and directive terms, knowing they must develop firm treatment plans for families and a sense of direction going forward. However, most parents do not want authoritarian guidance from providers. Instead, they seek collaborative relationships, in which all potential outcomes and treatment alternatives for their child are discussed.[7] They value openness and transparency during conversations, and wish to have their opinions and insights into their child's behavior respected and heard. This requirement for honesty is reflected by the AAP policy statement on patient-centered and family-centered care,[4] which urges pediatricians to share complete information with patients and their families in a manner that is supportive and unbiased.

However, families also expect clinicians to provide them with direction so that our young patients can receive appropriate therapies and access to care. There may be practical and ethical limits to discussing too much uncertainty with families, especially if doing so would overwhelm them, distract from the primary clinical problem, or add unnecessary time to treatment-urgent situations. Different families have different informational needs and may desire more or less participation in the shared decision-making process. Children must also be included in a way that is empowering and appropriate based on their developmental level. Thus, identifying each family's unique decisional needs, and recognizing the challenges of the clinical scenario at hand, can help clinicians filter and prioritize uncertainty for families while still engaging with them openly and honestly.

MANAGING UNCERTAINTY IN CLINICAL PRACTICE

Pediatricians must first recognize uncertainty before it can be addressed. Actively categorizing the components of a scenario as known and unknown can help identify where uncertainty is present.[8] It can then be further explored and classified according to existing conceptual frameworks[2,3] to determine which types can be reduced and which types must be tolerated. This classification informs pediatricians' approaches to history-taking and information-gathering and allows them to devise specific strategies for problem-solving.

Pediatricians must then acknowledge the extent of their comfort with uncertainty. Each clinician has a baseline tolerance that can change with time and experience, as seen with medical students as they become more advanced in their training.[3] However, pediatricians and other clinicians must still resist their natural tendencies toward too little or too much tolerance of uncertainty, as neither is desirable. Reis-Dennis and colleagues (2011) proposed three corrective skills or "virtues" that clinicians can use to balance their overall approach to uncertainty in any given scenario: courage, diligence, and curiosity.[5] Courage challenges clinicians to avoid oversimplification of ambiguous data and to embrace their discomfort with the unknown. Diligence motivates them to search the literature and/or to consult colleagues to avoid complacency. Finally, curiosity prompts them to engage with the scientific community to increase their overall knowledge and understanding of the unknown. Together, these virtues allow clinicians to approach uncertainty using a middle path that is characterized by a restlessness for clarity, yet an acceptance that some degree of uncertainty is unavoidable.

Finally, clinicians must recognize that uncertainty has a relational component. It is experienced by both clinicians and patients, although in different ways and to variable degrees.[2] Each party may or may not choose to reveal their experiences to the other. For example, a pediatrician may experience scientific uncertainty related to a child's diagnosis, yet refrain from discussing ambiguous clinical data with the family to avoid overwhelming them or generating unnecessary confusion. Similarly, a family may experience personal uncertainty about the impact of surgery on their child's quality of life, yet avoid discussing these issues with the clinician unless they are actively requested to do so.

Recognizing the balance of uncertainty between the two parties has significant implications for decision-making and may guide clinicians to shift the weight of decision-making toward either the clinician or the family based on the degree of uncertainty present and the stakes of the situation at hand.[9]

CASE ANALYSIS
Case 1

In this scenario, a community pediatrician is evaluating a young child for asthma, despite an absence of clear diagnostic information. The pediatrician may consider several diagnoses that could explain the boy's symptoms, including asthma, recurrent croup, and bronchiolitis. He or she must then navigate clinical data to arrive at the most appropriate diagnosis. However, interpreting these data can be complicated by insufficient information or confounding features such as the presence of wheezing but no clear improvement following treatment with a bronchodilator. Clinical data must be weighed carefully, and the diagnosis is ultimately subject to the pediatrician's personal judgment. Further complicating the picture are two future uncertainties, including the possibility that the boy could outgrow his symptoms and the possibility that an asthma diagnosis could restrict his ability to participate in competitive sports and to join the military.

When approaching this situation, the pediatrician might first ascertain the types of uncertainty present and determine what further clarification is possible. Because asthma is a disease of airflow limitation, uncertainty related to the diagnosis is usually resolved by obtaining pulmonary function testing. However, a 4-year-old child is too young to perform this test, and therefore, a diagnosis cannot be made solely on objective grounds. Accepting that some uncertainty must be tolerated, the pediatrician deliberates whether to observe the child, refer him to a specialist, or treat him empirically with inhaled steroids. He or she considers the degree of uncertainty present and the stakes of the decision at hand. Then, after recognizing his or her baseline tolerance of uncertainty, the pediatrician recommends a course of action that neither diagnoses prematurely nor delays treatment unnecessarily. In this particular scenario, the course of action could involve a time-limited trial of inhaled steroids over several months, with close monitoring of the boy's clinical response before deciding about a diagnosis of asthma.

Discussion with the family informs the chosen path, with the pediatrician engaging with them in a manner that is appropriate to their informational needs, and their desire to participate in shared decision-making.

Case 2

In our second case, the parents of a premature infant in the NICU face a decision about tracheostomy and home ventilation for their child. Choosing to proceed with home ventilation could facilitate an earlier discharge but may strain family relationships, cause undue financial burdens, and lead to social isolation. Choosing against it could either prolong the infant's hospitalization or lead to premature death. The parents' decision is complicated by the presence of numerous interrelated health problems that contribute to a variable prognosis for the child. Both the parents and the medical team must consider who could appropriately manage a technology-dependent child at home, whether the child will have access to a home nurse, and how the family will seek medical care when needed. Furthermore, the parents and medical team must consider the impact of tracheostomy and home ventilation on family life, relationships, the ability to travel, and the experience of the child who will be reliant on the technology. Similar to the first case, there are unknowns about the child's likelihood of improving over time, and whether there is potential for the tracheostomy tube to be removed in the future.

In this scenario, the clinician must help the family navigate the various treatment options in the presence of many uncertainties, some of which can be clarified while some of which cannot. For example, uncertainty about the child's overall outlook could be minimized by separating out her medical problems, and prognosticating about each individually. Issues related to personal uncertainty, however, such as the impact of tracheostomy on relationships and the infant's place within their family, can be explored but are more difficult to reduce. The stakes are extraordinarily high, and each party may have their own ideas about how to proceed.

Recognizing the relational nature of uncertainty, the clinician could lead a structured deliberation with the parents about the different treatment options, challenging them to consider the positive and negative consequences of each on the various aspects of their lives and eventually deferring to their choice given the high importance of the decision. Ultimately, the clinician must have the courage to embrace uncertainty with the family and guide their decision in a manner that aligns best with their values and goals.

SUMMARY

Various types of uncertainty are encountered in medicine, including those related to the limits of existing knowledge and unknowns about scientific, practical, and personal issues. Pediatricians may also experience uncertainties related to the role of families and the limited capacity of children in decision-making. Recognizing and identifying uncertainty is a critical first step in learning to manage it effectively. Pediatricians and other clinicians must then acknowledge their own comfort or discomfort and actively seek to avoid being too tolerant or too intolerant of its presence. Finally, pediatricians must understand that uncertainty is experienced both by families and by themselves as clinicians, and that the experience of uncertainty is balanced between the two parties. Choosing to filter and prioritize uncertainty together with families, while still allowing honest dialogue, maintains trust while maximizing transparency and collaboration.

CLINICS CARE POINTS

- Pediatricians must actively identify and categorize uncertainty in their practice in order to manage it effectively.

- Pediatricians should find balance between too much and too little tolerance of uncertainty in clinical practice.

- Pediatricians must recognize the interpersonal nature of uncertainty, actively discuss uncertainty with families, and adjust the weight of decision-making based on the degree of uncertainty present and the importance of the decision at hand.

DISCLOSURE

The authors declare that they have no conflicts of interest.

ACKNOWLEDGMENTS

The authors would like to acknowledge Sarah Louise Poynton, PhD, Johns Hopkins University School of Medicine, for her constructive critique of this article.

REFERENCES

1. Katz J. Why doctors don't disclose uncertainty. Hastings Cent Rep 1984;14(1): 35–44.
2. Han PK, Klein WM, Arora NK. Varieties of uncertainty in health care: a conceptual taxonomy. Med Decis Making 2011;31(6):828–38.

3. Fox RG. Training for Uncertainty. In: Merton RK, Reader GG, Kendall P, editors. The Student-physician: Introductory Studies in the Sociology of medical Education. Cambridge, MA: Harvard University Press; 1957. p. 207–42.

4. Committee on Hospital Care and Institute for patient- and family-centered care. Patient- and family-centered care and the pediatrician's role. Pediatrics 2012; 129(2):394–404.

5. Reis-Dennis S, Gerrity MS, Geller G. Tolerance for uncertainty and professional development: a normative analysis. J Gen Intern Med 2021;36(8):2408–13.

6. Ogden J, Fuks K, Gardner M, et al. Doctors expressions of uncertainty and patient confidence. Patient Educ Couns 2002;48(2):171–6.

7. Trocchia C, Singh P, Inglese C, et al. Navigating uncertainty in medicine with our families. Pediatrics 2023;151(4). e2022059783.

8. Boschetti F. A graphical representation of uncertainty in complex decision making. Emerg Complex Organ 2011;13:146–66.

9. Whitney SN. A new model of medical decisions: exploring the limits of shared decision making. Med Decis Making 2003;23(4):275–80.

Everyday Ethics in Ambulatory Pediatrics
Cases and Applications

Joseph A. Carrese, MD, MPH

KEYWORDS

- Ambulatory pediatrics • Everyday ethics • Outpatient ethics • Ethical analysis
- Ethical decision-making

KEY POINTS

- Ethics issues are commonly encountered in ambulatory pediatrics.
- It is important to have a strategy that systematically and thoroughly gathers, analyzes, and synthesizes information about ethics questions and concerns.
- It is critical to be aware of and understand the medical facts, patient/parent preferences, and larger contextual aspects of each case.
- Sources of information beyond the case may inform thinking and decision-making about the situation. Examples include relevant case law or statutory law; paradigm cases; articles in the literature; and professional guidelines.
- It is important to consider all possible stakeholders in any clinical scenario so their perspectives are accounted for.

INTRODUCTION

This article considers three clinical scenarios that might be encountered in ambulatory pediatric practice. The framework for ethical analysis presented by Dr Hughes in a separate article in this issue of the Pediatric Clinics of North America will be used to examine these clinical scenarios and demonstrate application of the framework. Of course, there is no shortage of clinical scenarios that could be chosen; ethics issues are commonly encountered in ambulatory pediatrics. The three scenarios presented are either especially challenging, relatively common or both.

Several possible strategies are available for analyzing cases that involve ethics questions and concerns. The approach described by Dr Hughes is one such strategy; it involves systematically and thoroughly gathering, analyzing, and synthesizing information. The expectation is that this process will lead to a better understanding of what is happening and related issues, a better analysis, and better recommendations.

Division of General Internal Medicine, Johns Hopkins Bayview Medical Center, Core Faculty, Johns Hopkins Berman Institute of Bioethics, Johns Hopkins University, Mason F. Lord Building, Center Tower, Suite 2300, 5200 Eastern Avenue, Baltimore, MD 21224, USA
E-mail address: jcarrese@jhmi.edu

Pediatr Clin N Am 71 (2024) 101–109
https://doi.org/10.1016/j.pcl.2023.08.005
0031-3955/24/© 2023 Elsevier Inc. All rights reserved.
pediatric.theclinics.com

Clinical Scenario 1

The parents of 9-year-old twins ask you to write a letter to be sent to the city housing authority stating they need to be considered for a larger Section 8 apartment to help them manage the boys' attention deficit-hyperactivity disorder (ADHD). Of note, the federal government's Section 8 rent voucher programs usually allots vouchers based on family size and income, but medical conditions may be considered. You know the boys are doing pretty well on standard doses of stimulant medication; they are also having success in school and their behavior toward each other has improved substantially. Both parents and the two boys currently live in a two-bedroom apartment.

What is the provider's concern? The provider is being asked to write a letter that will potentially include information that is not accurate, which would be dishonest. Being honest is widely recognized as a key component of common morality, and honesty is an essential element of building trust between providers and patients/parents. Being dishonest would violate a key personal and professional moral obligation of the provider.

Is this ethics? Yes. The ethical tension in this situation is between accommodating a parental request, thereby honoring their authority and autonomy versus the moral imperative to be truthful. In addition, considerations of fairness/justice are in play because the circumstances of this family are considered in the context of others in the community who may need and who might qualify for Section 8 housing, which is a limited resource.

Who are the stakeholders? Parents, child, provider, and other members of the community/public.

What are the facts of the case?

Medical condition. The standard management for ADHD includes pharmacologic and behavioral interventions. The major goals of therapy include improved relationships; better school performance; fewer disruptive behaviors; and enhanced self-esteem. We are told the boys are having success in school and their behavior toward each other has improved. It seems the current management plan is working pretty well.

Patient/parent perspective. The parents are requesting a different housing arrangement and they want that request accommodated. They indicate this request is to help them better manage their twins' ADHD. It is not known if that is the only factor involved in their request; perhaps another factor is involved or even the primary concern. One might consider interviewing the boys related to the parent's request, but given their age the primary moral agents and decision-makers in this situation are the parents.

Contextual features. It is possible that other factors the provider is unaware of, because they have not been articulated by the parents, are playing a role in this request, such as financial pressures or other issues in the family. Consideration might be given to probing this possibility with the parents. Part of the larger context is understanding what other housing options exist that the family might qualify for and being aware of the possibility that other families may have a stronger claim on the limited resource of Section 8 housing.

Are there other sources of information?

One other source of information that could be reviewed is the current policy and associated rules related to Section 8 housing. Specifically, what are the stated criteria for qualifying for this housing and does the family meet those criteria? If they do not, explaining that to the parents could be part of what is communicated to them when discussing why the letter they are requesting cannot be written, if that is what is decided.

What are the possible options and what action will be taken?
The main options in the situation are to write the letter being requested, and in doing so compromise one's honesty and integrity versus decline to write the letter and explain to the parents why you have made that decision. If you elect to not write the letter, you can still take steps to help address their request for different housing and potentially address the underlying reasons for their request.

Once an action is taken, what are the consequences?
The consequences, of course, depend on which action is pursued: if you decline to accommodate the parents' request, the relationship may be damaged and the parents may be upset that you did not help them out. On the other hand, if you decide to write the letter your integrity will be compromised, and your "standing" with the parents may be damaged because they will observe you being dishonest, even if it was in an effort to help them.

Discussion
In determining the appropriate response to this situation, it is worth considering the factors in favor and against accommodating the parents' request.[1] Factors in favor of accommodation might include parent/patient satisfaction; honoring parental authority and shared decision-making; advocating for the patients/parents; preserving the doctor–patient relationship and in turn the therapeutic alliance; and perhaps building trust and strengthening the relationship because you went to bat for them. Factors against accommodation might include damaging one's integrity by being dishonest; potential ramifications of including untrue information in a medical-legal document; loss of respect and in turn loss of trust by the parents because they observed you being dishonest, which in turn could damage the doctor–patient relationship; and concerns about justice/fairness to others.

To get a better understanding of what is else is going on and what else might be a factor in the parents' making this request one should consider exploring the nature of the problem that led to this request; specifically, are there any other factors besides ADHD? Depending on what is learned one can determine if there is any other way to meet the parents' goals that do not require you to be dishonest. The team social worker could be enlisted to help address these issues.

The following strategies for responding to what might be considered an inappropriate request should be considered: identify the issues as you see them and communicate your ethical obligations and concerns to the parents—honestly share with them the ethical bind this situation puts you in; explain to them your responsibilities to others (other patients/public; the profession); and be transparent no matter what you decide, explaining why you have made your choice.[1]

Clinical Scenario 2

Your patient is an 8 month-old girl with no significant past medical history. The parents tell you they plan to avoid the 1-year vaccinations. They have heard several stories about children developing fever, seizures, and myalgias after these vaccines. Worse, they have heard vaccination may diminish the body's ability to develop lifelong immunity. The family lives in a community where the vaccination rate for childhood vaccines is low at 84%. Ninety-two percent is considered adequate for herd immunity for the vaccines in question.

What is the provider's concern? The main concern in this situation is that a very well-established standard-of-care intervention (vaccinations) is being rejected by the parents of your very young patient.

Is this ethics? Yes. The central ethical tension in this situation is between benefitting the child and protecting her from harm versus respecting the authority of her parents to make decisions on her behalf.

Who are the stakeholders? Parents, child, provider, and community/public.

What are the facts of the case?
Medical condition. The medical issues in this situation are pretty straight forward: the goal of vaccination is to prevent significant downstream morbidity and mortality, both for individual patients and the community. The evidence base for approved vaccines is very strong and the risks are typically minor and more serious side effects are very rare. The risks of not getting vaccinated are considerable for both individual patients and, eventually, the community.

Patient/parent perspective. The parents in this situation believe the harms of recommended childhood vaccines outweigh any potential benefits. Their decision to decline the recommended vaccines is motivated by what they consider to be best for their child.

Contextual features. It is possible that other factors are playing a role in the parents' unwillingness to have their child vaccinated, for example, cultural and/or religious factors; information from the Internet or other sources; and beliefs of other family members or friends. An effort should be made to identify and explore any factors contributing to how they are approaching this issue.

Are there other sources of information?
Other sources of information in this scenario include the Advisory Committee on Immunization Practices and centers for disease control and prevention (CDC) recommended immunization schedules for children; the positions of professional associations such as the American Academy of Pediatrics (AAP); articles in the literature; and relevant state law and local school policy, to the extent they may have bearing on what is communicated to the parents about this issue.

What are the possible options and what action will be taken?
The main options are agreeing not to vaccinate the child for the time being but continuing to work with the parents to reach a mutual understanding and hopefully a way forward regarding vaccinations; proposing a modified vaccine schedule ("spreading out the shots") for the time being; or "firing" the family from your practice based primarily on concerns about the safety of other children in your practice.

Once an action is taken, what are the consequences?
It depends on which action is pursued: if you "fire" the family from your practice, the relationship ends and the opportunity to influence the parents and eventually treat the child is lost. The parents may eventually agree to vaccination if the relationship maintained and even if they do not you will continue to have the opportunity to address other health needs of the child.

Discussion
Vaccine hesitancy has become a major public health concern in recent years. The toll on individuals as well as communities is significant and increasing. A systematic review of this topic by Olson and colleagues addresses the key aspects of the problem,

including (but not limited to) the spectrum of vaccine acceptance; determinants of vaccine hesitancy; suggested communication interventions and strategies to address vaccine hesitancy; attention to the audience and the messenger for communication interventions; addressing misinformation and disinformation; and strategies for building trust.[2]

Some pediatric practices have taken the step of "firing" or dismissing families if they continue to decline recommended vaccinations, typically citing the safety and bests interests of other patients who may be vulnerable (eg, infants and sick kids) and at increased risk if infected.[3,4]

The AAPs position on this has evolved, from arguing against dismissing parents from the practice to acknowledging it as an option that can be legitimately considered but it is not a decision "that should be made lightly, nor should it be made without considering and respecting the reasons for the parents' point of view."[5]

One point is that this situation is an example of the broader category of patients/parents declining to do what is recommended by their treating clinician. Typically, adult patients with adequate decision-making capacity are given considerable latitude to decline what is recommended, as long as a good-faith effort has been made to ensure they have a sufficient understanding of the benefits of what is being recommended as well as the risks of declining. With adults, their right to be autonomous and self-determined can ultimately override the obligation to benefit them and protect them from harm. Similarly, parents are afforded considerable latitude regarding their authority to make decisions on behalf of their children, regarding what will and what would not be done. However, this authority is not absolute and, in some cases, may be appropriately overridden by concerns about the child's welfare. A key point is that a major part of any response to a patient/parent declining to do what is recommended is taking a step back and asking "Why?" It is important to inquire, explore, and potentially discover what is at the root of the decision to decline. If a specific reason is identified, this may create an opportunity for intervention, be if clarification, education (of patient/parent and/or provider), securing needed resources, and so on. One goal when what is being recommended is declined is to work to preserve the relationship to continue to have the opportunity to address other health concerns as well as the issue currently on the table.[6]

Although the scenario presented involves a very young child, other situations involving vaccines may occur with older children: older children may request vaccines but still need parental permission (eg, COVID); state laws may vary on this issue.[7] Alternatively, older children may decline vaccines their parents want them to get, which may be responded to differently depending on the age and maturity of the child and their development and emerging autonomy. Ideally, we would want the child's assent before proceeding with vaccination and may decide to honor the refusal of more mature adolescents.

Clinical Scenario 3

A physician believes contraception is a sin. He has communicated this to his patients, but his practice is located in a small town in rural western United States and he is the only provider who sees children. The next closest practice is more than 200 miles away. A 17-year-old patient comes to his office alone and asks him to prescribe contraception. She has become sexually active (against her parent's wishes) and wants very much to avoid pregnancy. She does not wish to be abstinent. She asks the physician to keep her visit and her request confidential.

What is the provider's concern? The physician seems to be primarily concerned about not violating his own, strongly held personal values/beliefs in the course of practicing medicine, and is therefore very unlikely to accommodate the patient's request. It is unknown based on the information presented, but it is presumed, which the physician will be at least somewhat troubled by deciding not to accommodate the patient's request for contraception, especially given the limited options available to the patient to get this prescription otherwise.

Is this ethics? Yes. In this scenario, the personal values and beliefs of the physician are in direct conflict with the patient's request to receive care that is legally available and considered standard of care in the United States—a request that a vast majority of other providers would accommodate.

Who are the stakeholders? Child, physician, community/public, and perhaps parents.

What are the facts of the case?

Medical condition. The medical facts in this scenario are straight forward: a sexually active 17-year-old girl seeks a prescription for contraception to prevent an unwanted pregnancy, and she requests that her parents not be told about the encounter. Although there are many contraception options and some are considered more effective than others, a broad category contraception is extremely effective in achieving the desired objective of preventing pregnancy. Also, the safety profile of Food and Drug Administration (FDA)-approved contraception options is very good.

Patient/parental perspective. This 17 year old has requested a prescription for contraception to prevent an unwanted pregnancy, and she requests that her parents not be told about the encounter. Although she is not yet 18-year-old and therefore does not have the same status in terms of providing legally recognized consent if she were 18, in most jurisdictions in the US adolescents do have a right under state law to make their own decisions about treatment for reproductive health issues (and other health-related issues as well, such as sexually transmitted infections (STIs), substance use; and mental health issues). Also, with rare exception, such treatment can proceed confidentially, without parental notification. In this scenario, the patient has elected to exercise her right to seek treatment confidentially.

Of course, it is clear from what we are told in the scenario that her parents would not agree with her being sexually active and presumably would also not agree with her getting a prescription for contraception.

Contextual features. The main contextual feature in this scenario is the physician's views about the use of contraception being sinful. Presumably, this view is directly related to his particular religious tradition and his understanding of what that tradition holds about contraception use. Other contextual factors include the patient's parents and their views about her being sexually active and the geographic setting of the scenario: rural United States with very limited options for the 17-year-old patient in terms of securing the contraception prescription other than from this physician.

Are there other sources of information?

Legal information and the ethics literature on this topic are extensive. The relevant laws vary by state regarding what rights adolescents have in terms of making decisions about their own care without parental notification (eg, regarding reproductive, mental health, and substance use) and regarding when parents must be involved and in turn grant permission (consent) for medical care for their child. Opinion 1.1.7 ("Physician Exercise of Conscience) of the AMA Code of medical ethics addresses the issues in play in this clinical scenario in depth and thoughtfully.[8]

What are the possible options and what action will be taken?
It seems very likely, based on the information provided in the scenario, that the physician will adopt a strict "no" stance and would not prescribe the requested contraception. The physician probably also would not facilitate an alternative solution, because doing so would be regarded as being complicit in sinful behavior. It is possible the physician would not prescribe but will try to facilitate a solution for the patient (seen as a minimum requirement by many). A final option is that the physician will decide, after careful consideration of the circumstances, to prescribe a contraceptive treatment even though doing so is against his personal beliefs.

Once an action is taken, what are the consequences?
If the physician declines to prescribe the requested contraception, this may end the relationship with this patient. If the patient is unsuccessful in securing a prescription for contraception and she remains sexually active an unwanted pregnancy may result. It is possible the physician would not prescribe the contraception but will try to help facilitate a solution, in which the relationship may be preserved for future encounters. If the physician decides to prescribe the contraception, this will also likely preserve the relationship, but it may result in damage to the physician's sense of integrity as it relates to his personal values and moral code.

Discussion
As noted earlier, the central ethical tension in this scenario is between a health care provider exercising their right to not provide information or care that violates their deeply held values/beliefs (their "right of conscience") versus a patient expecting and receiving legally permitted and effective standard of care.

There is a very extensive literature on this topic, covering the full range of views. At one end of the continuum, some investigators argue you should not be practicing medicine if you are unwilling to accommodate patient requests for legally available, standard-of-care treatment.[9] In this same vein, the investigators have criticized doctors who claim "an unfettered right to personal autonomy while holding monopolistic control over a public good."[10] At the other end of the continuum, some investigators argue that providers should have a robust right of conscience,[11] and in some states, this view has been codified in law: "For example, the Illinois Health Care Right of Conscience Act protects a health care provider from all liability or discrimination that might result as a consequence of 'his or her refusal to perform, assist, counsel, suggest, recommend, refer or participate in any way in any particular form of health care service which is contrary to the conscience of such physician or health care personnel.'"[12]

A middle ground is recognizing that although a right of conscience is something all of us might want to invoke in certain, hopefully rare circumstances (eg, a military physician being ordered to place a feeding tube over and against the objections of a prisoner on hunger strike[13]), for the most part we expect providers to respect and honor their patients' requests for legally permitted and effective health care, despite the provider's personal values/views.

In the scenario presented if the physician does not accommodate the patient's request for a prescription for contraception because of his own personal religious values that has the effect in this very rural community (with no other provider nearby) of imposing the physician's moral values on the community, they are charged with caring for. In geographic areas with more options (eg, cities, suburban communities), we can more easily imagine a solution that allows the provider to hold the line on not violating their personal values (by not prescribing), but at the same time, making sure that the 17-year-old patient is connected with a provider who will prescribe this medication in a timely fashion.

The broader implications of this issue include the acceptability of providers having inflexible personal values/views that interfere with their ability to practice medicine in a very diverse society, where many patients/families may not share those values/views. One legitimate worry about clinicians invoking right of conscience is the extent to which patients, especially vulnerable patients, will lose access to essential medical care.[14]

Arguably being self-aware, embracing cultural humility and having a flexible mindset will serve providers and their patients well. Finally, disclosure and transparency about any restrictions in one's practice related to one's personal values is recommended, as is dialogue and negotiation in trying to arrive at a mutually acceptable solution that avoids violating either party's values, if that is possible.

DISCLOSURE

The author has nothing to disclose.

REFERENCES

1. Green MJ. Inappropriate requests for medical exemptions and privileges. In: Sugarman J, editor. Ethics in primary care. New York: McGraw-Hill, Health Professions Division; 2000. p. 13–25.
2. Olsen O, Berry C, Kumar N. Addressing Parental Vaccine Hesitancy towards Childhood Vaccines in the United States: A Systematic Literature Review of Communication Interventions and Strategies. Vaccines (Basel) 2020; 8(4):590.
3. O'Leary ST, Cataldi JR, Lindley MC. Policies Among US Pediatricians for Dismissing Patients for Delaying or Refusing Vaccination. JAMA 2020;324(11): 1105–7.
4. Halperin B, Melnychuk R, DownieJ, et al. When is it permissible to dismiss a family who refuses vaccines? Legal, ethical and public health perspectives. Paediatr Child Health 2007;12(10):843–5.
5. Edwards KM, Hackell JM. the Committee on Infectious Diseases, the Committee on Practice and Ambulatory Medicine. Countering vaccine hesitancy. Pediatrics 2016;138(3):e20162146.
6. Carrese J. Responding to Rejection. February 2023. [Link to article: Responding to Rejection - CLOSLER - CLOSLER.]
7. State Parental Consent Laws for COVID-19 Vaccination. In: Kaiser Family Foundation. 2021. Available at: https://www.kff.org/other/state-indicator/state-parental-consent-laws-for-covid-19.vaccination/?currentTimeframe=0&sortModel=%7B%22colId%22:%22Location%22,%22sort%22:%22asc%22%7D. Accessed April 6, 2023.
8. Opinion 1.1.7, Physician Exercise of Conscience in Responsibilities of Physician and Patients in Opinions on Patient-Physician Relationships, AMA Code of Medical Ethics Opinions.
9. Savulescu J. Conscientious Objection in Medicine. Br Med J (Clin Res Ed) 2006; 332:294–7.
10. Charo RA. The celestial fire of conscience- refusing to deliver medical care. N Engl J Med 2005;352:2471–3.

11. Sulmasy DP. Professional Judgment, and the Discretionary Space of the Physician. Camb Q Healthc Ethics 2017;26(1):18–31.
12. Health Care Right of Conscience Act, 745 Ill. Comp. Stat. § 70/1-14.
13. Crosby SS, Apovian CM, Grodin MA. Hunger Strikes, Force-feeding, and Physicians' Responsibilities. JAMA 2007;298(5):563–6.
14. Gostin L. The "Conscience" Rule: How Will It Affect Patients' Access to Health Services? JAMA 2019;321(22):2152–3.

Moving?

Make sure your subscription moves with you!

To notify us of your new address, find your **Clinics Account Number** (located on your mailing label above your name), and contact customer service at:

Email: journalscustomerservice-usa@elsevier.com

800-654-2452 (subscribers in the U.S. & Canada)
314-447-8871 (subscribers outside of the U.S. & Canada)

Fax number: 314-447-8029

Elsevier Health Sciences Division
Subscription Customer Service
3251 Riverport Lane
Maryland Heights, MO 63043

*To ensure uninterrupted delivery of your subscription, please notify us at least 4 weeks in advance of move.

Printed and bound by CPI Group (UK) Ltd, Croydon, CR0 4YY

03/10/2024

01040473-0010